D0023336

Your Child Does *Not* Have Bipolar Disorder

Recent Titles in Childhood in America

Your Child Does *Not* Have Bipolar Disorder

How Bad Science and Good Public Relations Created the Diagnosis

STUART L. KAPLAN, MD

Childhood in America
Sharna Olfman, Series Editor

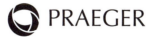

AN IMPRINT OF ABC-CLIO, LLC
Santa Barbara, California • Denver, Colorado • Oxford, England

Library of Congress Cataloging-in-Publication Data

Kaplan, Stuart L.
    Your child does not have bipolar disorder : how bad science and good public relations created the diagnosis / Stuart L. Kaplan.
        p. cm. — (Childhood in America)
    Includes bibliographical references and index.
    ISBN 978-0-313-38134-8 (hard copy : alk. paper) — ISBN 978-0-313-38135-5 (ebook)
1. Manic-depressive illness in children—Popular works. I. Title. II. Series.
    RJ506.D4K37   2011
    618.92'895—dc22   2010047612

ISBN: 978-0-313-38134-8
EISBN: 978-0-313-38135-5

15 14 13 12 11   1 2 3 4 5

This book is also available on the World Wide Web as an eBook.

Visit www.abc-clio.com for details.

Praeger
An Imprint of ABC-CLIO, LLC

ABC-CLIO, LLC
130 Cremona Drive, P.O. Box 1911
Santa Barbara, California 93116-1911

This book is printed on acid-free paper (∞)

Manufactured in the United States of America

To Joan Kaplan, my wife and soul mate, and to
Lawrence Kaplan, my son and good friend

In memory of my father, mother, and brother:
Leonard Kaplan, Anne Kaplan, and Philip B. Kaplan

Contents

Acknowledgments

I am grateful to Dr. Joan Kaplan, Sarah Manges, Naomi Busner, and Philip Busner for their editorial assistance and support. I also wish to thank Dr. Sharna Olfman for including this book in her important series, Childhood in America. Finally, I thank Dr. Walter Kaplan and Benita Kaplan for their affectionate support throughout the preparation of the book.

Introduction

In the autumn of 1993 I attended a workshop on bipolar disorder in prepubertal children at the annual meeting of the American Academy of Child and Adolescent Psychiatry. About 10 psychiatrists attended the workshop, which was held in a small, poorly lit room. Only one or two of the doctors present reported actually having seen a prepubertal child with bipolar disorder, but we all agreed to keep our eyes open for other sightings. After the meeting, I returned home to meet with the staff of the large psychiatric inpatient unit I ran for children ages 13 and younger. I asked if anyone on staff had diagnosed a child patient with bipolar disorder. The staff reported that they had never seen such a child.

Approximately three years later, I attended another session about bipolar disorder in prepubertal children at the American Academy of Child and Adolescent Psychiatry annual meeting. This session was held in a huge ballroom beneath a gleaming chandelier, and there were several hundred child psychiatrists in attendance, all of them buzzing with excitement. This was, for me, the first tangible evidence of the tidal wave of unwarranted enthusiasm that was about to engulf the public and the profession for the still relatively new diagnosis of pediatric bipolar disorder.

In less than a decade, from roughly 1994 to 2003, the diagnosis and treatment of bipolar disorder in children and adolescents underwent a dramatic transformation. Before 1995, bipolar disorder was rarely diagnosed in children and adolescents; today nearly one-third of all children and adolescents discharged from child psychiatric hospitals have been diagnosed with bipolar disorder and are treated accordingly (Blader & Carlson, 2007). The rise of outpatient office visits for children and adolescents with bipolar disorder has increased forty-fold, from 20,000 in 1994–1995 to 800,000 in 2002–2003 (Moreno et al., 2007).

Your Child Does Not *Have Bipolar Disorder* will examine this phenomenon through a variety of lenses. I will draw heavily on my 40 years of experience as a clinician, researcher, and professor of child psychiatry and will make the argument that bipolar disorder in children and many adolescents is incorrectly diagnosed and incorrectly treated. I will discuss the events that precipitated the dramatic increase in the diagnosis, present the evidence against the diagnosis, and describe effective alternative diagnostic and treatment approaches for the serious difficulties these children do exhibit.

Psychiatry, like all branches of medicine, is expected to be based on science. Research is ongoing, and treatment methodology is updated regularly. This, in part, is what makes the dramatic rise in this particular diagnosis so disturbing: It is not based on scientific evidence. It does not reflect any new discovery or insight about the etiology or treatment of the disorder. In fact, the opposite seems to be the case: the scientific evidence *against* the existence of child bipolar disorder is so strong that it is difficult to imagine how it has gained the endorsement of anyone in the scientific community.

Although these children do not have bipolar disorder, they are seriously disturbed. They often have behavior problems at home and at school. They are disrespectful to their teachers, they run around in school hallways, and they are unable to sit still in class or concentrate on schoolwork. Prone to violent outbursts, they may hit other children and get in trouble for fighting. In more serious cases, they may be in and out of child psychiatric units and may end up in juvenile detention centers. Their home lives may be chaotic. Their parents are often exhausted and sometimes feel hopeless. These are children like Victoria, an 11-year-old whose history of violent temper tantrums included breaking her father's ankle with an iron bar, and Shanice, age 10, whose family came to see me after her ninth hospitalization for bipolar disorder.

For children such as these and their families, a misdiagnosis of bipolar disorder can have devastating consequences. Such children are regularly prescribed medications that, although effective in adults with bipolar disorder, are not effective in children, are laden with risk, and have unwelcome side effects.

Because these children are being treated for something they don't have, they often don't get treated for what they do have. It is well established that 60% to 90% of children who have been diagnosed with bipolar disorder also have attention deficit hyperactivity disorder (ADHD) (Singh, DelBello, Kowatch, & Strakowski, 2006). It has also been well chronicled that, dosed correctly, 80% of children with ADHD respond favorably and dramatically to stimulant medication (Greenhill et al., 2002). Unfortunately, those who champion the cause of bipolar disorder in childhood routinely warn against the medication treatment of ADHD. Instead they have insisted, with almost no evidence, that such treatment will lead to a dramatic worsening of the bipolar disorder. Thus, the one class of medication that might be most helpful is frequently withheld.

It is my hope that this book will facilitate the reevaluation of the diagnosis and treatment of many children now misdiagnosed as having bipolar disorder.

Although I can't know without meeting you and your child that your child does not have bipolar disorder, I have interviewed thousands of psychiatrically disturbed children under 13 years of age and have never found a child I believed actually had this diagnosis. Therefore it is highly likely that were I to examine your child, I also would conclude that your child does not have bipolar disorder.

This book is an argument against the diagnosis of bipolar disorder in childhood. It is directed at parents, mental health professionals, and anyone interested in major issues in contemporary child psychiatry. My main argument is simplified by confining it to prepubertal children initially, but the argument is broadened later to include adolescents.

The book is divided into three parts. Part I consists of a critique of the bipolar disorder diagnosis among children and adolescents as well as a critique of the studies that have attempted to support the diagnosis. Some of the social and cultural forces that have influenced the rapid and wide-scale adoption of the pediatric bipolar disorder diagnosis are explored. Part II considers the medications that have been involved in the treatment of children and adolescents misdiagnosed with bipolar disorder. Part III provides direct advice for parents.

REFERENCES

Blader, J.C., & Carlson, G.A. (2007). Increased rates of bipolar disorder diagnoses among U.S. child, adolescent, and adult inpatients, 1996–2004. *Biol Psychiatry, 62*(2), 107–114.

PART I

Critique of Pediatric Bipolar Disorder

misdiagnosed as having it. These children will be described in the next chapter.

ADULT BIPOLAR DISORDER

Bipolar disorder, once known as "manic-depressive illness," is characterized by cycles in which a patient rotates between two extremes, or poles, of feeling states: depression and mania. Mania is a necessary component of the diagnosis of bipolar disorder: without a distinct period of mania, the diagnosis cannot be made. In order to appreciate fully what is meant by mania, it may be helpful to understand some of the common behaviors and experiences associated with the condition as it appears to clinicians and patients (Goodwin & Jamison, 2007).

Often, mania begins with a pleasant feeling of happiness. The patients are more pleased than usual with themselves and their capabilities. They begin to talk more loudly and rapidly. They become more active physically and mentally, are able to think more quickly, and accomplish much more than usual with little sense of effort. They have increasingly ambitious ideas about projects at home and work, and everything begins to seem possible. The world may appear fresher and brighter, and the patients' own emotional responses to the world and other people may seem heightened. They become excited about their lives and their activities. Their enjoyment in talking with people increases, and they quickly develop a wider circle of friends. They require less sleep. As the mania develops, they crave more frequent sexual activity and more sexual partners. They believe that they are thinking more quickly and accomplishing more in a reduced amount of time. In the background of these pleasant feelings, irritability may break through as they become less able to wait patiently for the slowness of other people.

This level of mania is known as "hypomania" and is extremely pleasant for patients; they have no desire to give it up. They do not experience themselves as mentally ill; instead, they experience themselves as having a marked increase in productivity, creativity, and happiness.

This is not how they are experienced by others. In the memoir *An Unquiet Mind* by Kay Jamison, PhD—a psychologist who also suffers from bipolar disorder—this was described poignantly (Jamison, 2007). As a female first-year graduate student, Jamison attended a reception for new students given by her dean. At the party she found herself to be charming and witty. She believed that she had managed to interest other faculty members in several of her projects and that she had captivated many senior department members with her affability and charm. Many months after the party, she learned that others regarded her behavior quite differently. She had been seen as having worn inappropriate, sexually provocative clothing, having had poorly applied, smeary makeup, and as having talked loudly and fast. Most people at the party, she was told, had had a difficult time understanding her.

Hypomanic patients are recognized by their friends and family as behaving differently from their usual selves, and the difference does not always win social approval. The patients believe that there is nothing wrong with them and shrug off suggestions that they seek help. They refuse to recognize the overexcited, loud, intrusive quality of their behavior. The pleasure they experience in this state leaves most hypomanic patients reluctant to seek or accept treatment.

There is much that is enviable about hypomanic states. Hypomanic patients are active, energetic, tireless, personable, intensely committed to work, ambitious, and sexually active, and they derive great joy from life. Jamison (2004) has argued persuasively that many of mankind's greatest accomplishments in poetry, music, and other areas have been created by individuals in hypomanic or closely related states.

The bliss of the hypomanic state faces many threats. The patient's hypomania may intensify and result in manic symptoms that impair rather than enhance functioning. Shifting from a hypomanic state to a manic state often leads to patients becoming more aggressive, irritable, and intolerant of what they perceive to be others' shortcomings. Becoming less inhibited, they may become loud, rude, and may curse and engage in physical fights. They speak incessantly and become enraged if others try to interrupt or redirect a conversation. They make poor decisions about handling their sex lives that can get them into a variety of difficulties with spouses and acquaintances. Money is spent with increasing recklessness, and extravagant purchases may be made that are not affordable. A typical complaint from a family with a manic breadwinner is the patient bringing home a luxury car such as a Rolls Royce that the family can ill afford. Ambitious business plans become increasingly far-fetched. With great excitement patients may contact a large number of investors to put up money for unrealistic business deals. One of the ironies of patients in this state is that they can organize themselves to be very persuasive and may actually convince others to invest in their projects. The patients think quickly, speak loudly, and are intrusive. They can sleep as little as three hours per night, sometimes less, and still feel rested. The manic patients' self-esteem and self-regard are extremely high.

The patients' mania may continue to evolve until they become psychotic. Psychotic symptoms can include delusions (fixed, false beliefs) and hallucinations (seeing and hearing things that are not present). The delusions developed by many manic patients are often paranoid, meaning that they sometimes believe that people are out to hurt them or are plotting against them. They may also develop grandiose delusions—believing themselves to be religious or mythological figures or believing that they possess special powers or importance.

Sometimes the behaviors are disruptive to the extent of requiring hospitalization. This was the case with Ms. Jones, a 20-year-old single woman whom I met several days after she was discharged from her first psychiatric hospitalization for bipolar disorder. She had been brought to the emergency room by her supervisor at work, who was concerned about her rapid, incoherent, loud speech, and disheveled appearance. At the hospital she was interviewed by a psychiatrist who immediately recognized her as acutely manic and hospitalized her.

A month earlier, Ms. Jones had begun working in a hospital laboratory after completing a year-long laboratory technician program. Within a week, she began to make complaints to the supervisor about the poor work habits of her colleagues, claiming that they were lazy and indifferent to laboratory procedures. At home her behavior had become quite bizarre. She told her boyfriend that she had been called by God to become a doctor and heal people in faraway lands. She told him that she believed she was destined to make major medical discoveries. She began looking for medical schools on the Internet and told her boyfriend that she felt certain they would accept her. Although she had never been particularly interested in her studies, she began to call for applications to Ivy League colleges for "pre-med" studies in anticipation of applying to medical school. She became enraged frequently and would destroy objects in the house if her boyfriend or others questioned her ability to attend medical school. Along with her medical school plans, she enrolled in a Bible study group and began staying up all night reading sections of the Bible aloud. She believed that it was her calling to become a doctor and do medical missionary work. She slept a total of one or two hours a night without feeling tired. She began calling acquaintances and relatives at odd hours demanding money to pursue her goal of becoming a medical missionary. On the day she was hospitalized, Ms. Jones had spoken to her supervisor at work to announce that she needed a leave of absence so she could pursue her goal of becoming a medical missionary.

While in the hospital, Ms. Jones slept little and read the Bible incessantly. She came to believe that she had the power to help the other patients on the unit by touching them on the back and on the chest, which she described as a biblical prescription for healing the sick. She sang hymns six to seven hours a day and organized several other patients to join her in singing. She continued to believe that she did not have bipolar disorder, though she did not refuse the medication prescribed during her hospital stay. She was significantly better and ready for discharge within two weeks. Fear of rehospitalization and her fear of losing her boyfriend and job prompted her to continue to take her prescribed medication and to attend therapy appointments regularly. She continued to improve and was able to resume employment at the hospital laboratory.

Patients in severely manic states barely sleep, may barely eat, and as their judgment deteriorates, put others as well as themselves at risk. Typically, manic patients refuse treatment and cannot be controlled. They are overactive and angry, and it is not unusual for severely manic patients to be brought in to an emergency room by the police and then psychiatrically hospitalized against their will. Manic patients are very often enraged at confinement of their activities to an inpatient psychiatric unit and may become violent.

In the less severe stages of mania, patients may be able to fake an absence of mental illness. This is most often seen when families bring manic relatives for evaluation to psychiatric hospitalization and the patients do not wish to be hospitalized. The patients may behave very reasonably during the psychiatric evaluation to avoid hospitalization but then resume their bizarre behaviors immediately following the psychiatric interview.

The opposite is possible as well. A group of women with long-standing bipolar disorder living in a home for the chronically mentally ill lost the heat in the home in the middle of a bitterly cold winter. At their own request, they were brought by the police to a psychiatric emergency room where, seen individually, they seemed agitated and psychotic. They wanted to be admitted to the psychiatric hospital, and they were. Immediately after they were admitted, all calmed considerably and talked rationally among themselves amiably and at great length. The agitation prior to admission may have been feigned to secure admission to the warmth of the heated psychiatric unit.

Both mania and hypomania typically end in a crushing, painful depression. Patients lose their capacity to enjoy life, become despondent, suffer feelings of intense guilt, and often contemplate suicide.

An episode of depression that shortly follows an obvious, recognized manic episode is easily diagnosed as a depressed phase of bipolar disorder. If the bipolar disorder begins as depression, however, without a preceding hypomanic or manic episode, it is not possible to recognize the depression as part of bipolar disorder; the diagnosis of bipolar disorder requires an episode of mania or hypomania. Further complicating the task of diagnosing bipolar disorder, the patient may not recognize having had a hypomanic phase in the past and may seek treatment only after the appearance of the depression. During a first depressive episode, the patient may deny any previous symptoms of hypomania. It is only the psychological pain of the depression that leads him or her to seek help.

Bipolar disorder patients often cycle from mania to depression and back to mania again; between these manic or depressed episodes are apparently normal periods of functioning. Most of the patients (90%) who have had one episode are likely to have another "mood swing" or episode. These subsequent mood swings are often preventable with medication if the patient agrees to take it; bipolar disorder patients who are early in the course of their illness may find it difficult to believe that they continue to have the illness and continue to require medication.

Although bipolar disorder might present itself in a variety of ways, all cases share a common set of symptoms. In order for a diagnosis to be made certain criteria must be met. These criteria, which are listed in the *DSM-IV*, are not ambiguous: they are described explicitly and with great care.

The argument against the diagnosis of pediatric bipolar disorder is that pediatric bipolar disorder does not meet the *DSM-IV* criteria for bipolar disorder. In fact, the disorder in children looks nothing like the disorder in adults. Before we can attempt a detailed comparison of the two, however, it will be helpful to gain some understanding of the *DSM* system of psychiatric diagnosis and to see how this system works in diagnosing bipolar disorder.

THE *DSM* SYSTEM

The resolution of any dispute about the diagnosis of a psychiatric disorder must begin by consulting the authoritative description of psychiatric diagnoses: the *DSM-IV* of the American Psychiatric Association. "DSM" stands for *Diagnostic Statistical Manual*, and "IV" stands for the fourth edition (American Psychiatric Association, 2000).

There is a new edition of this manual published about every 10 years, and often there are minor revisions every 5 years. The manual is based largely on the recommendations of committees of experts in every diagnostic area who review the available published research studies and any known unpublished data in their areas of expertise. The diagnostic criteria are subject to lengthy critical discussions, and contributions outside the committee structure are also sought from the larger professional and consumer public. As part of the *DSM* process, the criteria are field tested with actual patients to ensure that professionals can use them with relative ease to diagnose patients. In these so-called field trials, the ability of mental health professionals to achieve agreement about the diagnosis is carefully studied.

The *DSM-IV* criteria are easily observable or easily obtained from patient report. These criteria are symptom based and in general do not refer to any causes or theories about illnesses. If a patient has the symptomatic criteria for the illness, he or she has the psychiatric illness. The *DSM-IV* system is based on the humbling truth that the cause of mental illness remains unknown.

The criteria outlined in the *DSM-IV* tend to facilitate a patient receiving the same diagnosis regardless of where he or she is receiving care. Before *DSM-IV* (and its predecessor, *DSM-III*, published in 1980) a patient diagnosed as having schizophrenia at one hospital might receive a different diagnosis at another hospital because of differences in theoretical orientations at the two hospitals. By having observable objective criteria for the diagnosis of mental illness, the *DSM-III* and *DSM-IV* systems minimized these discrepancies between institutions.

Criticisms of *DSM-IV* are plentiful but generally misguided. For example, *DSM-IV* uses specific symptoms to define a psychiatric illness. These symptoms must be asked about and noted to be present or absent. This has led to the complaint that the *DSM-IV* is dehumanizing to patients in that it minimizes or ignores the patients' life stories. John Sadler, MD, a professor and distinguished philosopher of psychiatry, suggested that talking only about symptoms pushes both the professional and the patient to become machine-like, with the professional almost robotically asking *DSM-IV* questions and the patient replying in a similar fashion (Sadler, 2009). Making a related point, David Healy, MD, a distinguished psychiatrist and author, noted that the *DSM* system promotes informational reductionism. By attending only to symptoms and ignoring the patients' history and current problems, he argued, the *DSM* system reduces the amount of information the mental health professional learns about the patient (Healy, 2009).

Although some users of *DSM-IV* may operate in such a fashion, there is nothing in *DSM-IV* that prohibits exploration of the patients' history, current problems, or any other aspect of the patient. And the standards of care of the various professions—such as the American Academy of Child and Adolescent Psychiatry practice parameters for child psychiatric evaluation—demand that professionals take account of these issues. A good psychiatric diagnostician uses the *DSM-IV* symptoms as a portal into important aspects of a patient's life experience.

A third criticism of the *DSM-IV* concerns its major assumption that psychiatric illness is categorical. This means that a patient either has the illness or does not have it, with little in between. If the criteria are met, the patient has the illness; if the criteria are not met, the patient does not have the illness. The categorical approach of *DSM-IV* contrasts with a "spectrum approach" to illness that views most patients as having parts of many illnesses in different degrees. The benefit of the categorical approach to diagnosis is that it has served as an important barrier to the unwarranted proliferation of labeling people ill who are not.

Finally, and directly related to child mental health, is the criticism that *DSM-IV* lacks a developmental approach. It is claimed that differences between psychiatric illness in children and adults are ignored and differences in psychological development at different ages are treated as if they do not exist. It is true that *DSM-IV* criteria do largely ignore differences between children and adults; *DSM-IV* considers the disorders to be isomorphic (the same criteria apply to children and adults). This may seem to be a simplistic approach to the diagnosis of psychiatric disorders in children and adolescents, but it has been surprisingly effective. For example, prior to *DSM-III*, children and adolescents were not believed to have symptoms of depression. With the application of the *DSM-III* adult symptoms of depression to children and adolescents, however, this population was unexpectedly demonstrated for the first time to have adult symptoms of depressive illness. The opposite has been found as well. Attention deficit hyperactivity disorder (ADHD), long believed to be only a disorder of childhood and adolescence, has been found in adults as well using the *DSM-IV* criteria for the disorder. Adults respond equally well to medications routinely used in children for ADHD.

Regardless of the value of these criticisms, *DSM-IV* criteria serve as the accepted diagnostic criteria of psychiatric illness by clinicians, psychiatric researchers, insurance companies, the American legal system, the Food and Drug Administration, and the vast majority of mental health service providers in the United States.

For all *DSM-IV* diagnoses, there is a list of criteria that must be met in order to have the diagnosis. The "A" criterion is usually considered to be the most important or defining criterion of the syndrome. As can be seen from the list of criteria for a manic episode in Table 1.1, the "A" criterion of one week's duration of expansive or elevated mood can be substituted with irritability and can be shortened to less than one week if the patient is hospitalized. The "B" criterion requires the simultaneous presence of three of the seven listed symptoms—four if the mood is irritable. The "C" criterion reminds the diagnostician that all of the symptoms must be consistent with mania; a manic episode that has all the symptoms of mania plus mixes in symptoms of depression is known as "mixed"—another form of a manic episode. The "D" criterion refers to impairment, which means that the symptoms must interfere with the patient's life. Finally, the "E" criterion reminds the diagnostician that, like most *DSM-IV* diagnoses, a psychiatric diagnosis

TABLE 1.1. DSM-IV Criteria for Manic Episode

A. A distinct period of abnormally and persistently elevated, expansive, or irritable mood, lasting at least 1 week (or any duration if hospitalization is necessary).

B. During the period of mood disturbance, three (or more) of the following symptoms have persisted (four if the mood is only irritable) and have been present to a significant degree:
    (1) inflated self-esteem or grandiosity
    (2) decreased need for sleep (e.g., feels rested after only 3 hours of sleep)
    (3) more talkative than usual or pressure to keep talking
    (4) flight of ideas or subjective experience that thoughts are racing
    (5) distractibility (i.e., attention too easily drawn to unimportant or irrelevant external stimuli)
    (6) increase in goal-directed activity (either socially, at work or school, or sexually) or psychomotor agitation
    (7) excessive involvement in pleasurable activities that have a high potential for painful consequences (e.g., engaging in unrestrained buying sprees, sexual indiscretions, or foolish business investments)

C. The symptoms do not meet criteria for a Mixed Episode

D. The mood disturbance is sufficiently severe to cause marked impairment in occupational functioning or in usual social activities or relationships with others, or to necessitate hospitalization to prevent harm to self or others, or there are psychotic features.

E. The symptoms are not due to the direct physiological effects of a substance (e.g., a drug of abuse, a medication, or other treatment) or a general medical condition (e.g., hyperthyroidism).

(Reprinted with permission from the *Diagnostic and Statistical Manual of Mental Disorders, Fourth Edition*, Text Revision [Copyright 2000]. American Psychiatric Association.)

is not permitted if the condition is due to a medical illness or some other biological cause such as medication or drugs.

Most of these criteria were illustrated in the first portion of this chapter, but there remains one critical point that will be especially relevant going forward: mania, by definition, is not a chronic condition, and the patient cannot have been this way his or her entire life. The "A" criterion specifies "A *distinct* period . . ." (emphasis added). When a patient is in a manic state, a different way of behaving and thinking emerges that is largely unrelated to the patient's previous behavior. Of necessity, the seven listed symptoms of mania (of which three must be present for the diagnosis) must have developed with the onset of the "*distinct* period." They were not present before the onset of the manic episode. Only if the patient first becomes overactive and distracted with the onset of elevated mood (euphoria) do the symptoms count toward a

diagnosis of mania. If the patient has always been overactive and distracted, the symptoms do *not* count toward a diagnosis of mania. *Distinct* refers to "different from the patient's usually functioning."

The "A" criterion of mania demands a period of *"persistently elevated,
expansive, or irritable mood"* (emphasis added). Even if the diagnosis of
mania is based on irritability rather than euphoria, the irritability must
represent a distinct period—clearly different from the person's usual
behavior. The elevated or expansive mood is not the happiness of a
birthday or of Christmas. Instead, this lasts for at least a week and
meets the criteria for the symptoms as described in the "B" criteria.
Only after the patient has met the criteria for a manic episode can the
DSM-IV diagnosis of bipolar disorder be considered.

There are many different forms of *DSM-IV* bipolar disorder, and it
is useful to distinguish among some of them. "Bipolar I disorder, single manic episode," is given to a patient who has had a single manic
episode but has never had a depressive episode. "Bipolar I disorder,
most recent episode manic," requires a present or past manic episode
with a past history of at least one other manic episode. If there were
depressed or mixed (manic plus depressed) episodes, the most recent
past episode must have been manic. "Bipolar I disorder, most recent
episode depressed," requires the occurrence of at least one past manic
episode, but the most recent episode the patient experienced must
have been a depressive episode. The *DSM-IV* also recognizes "bipolar II disorder," which requires at least one "hypomanic" episode and
one or more depressive episodes. A hypomanic episode is similar to a
manic episode but is less severe.

When a disorder does not meet all the necessary criteria, *DSM-IV*
allows for the label "not otherwise specified" (NOS). This means that
the patient, by definition, does not meet the full criteria of the disorder, but *DSM-IV* allows the diagnostician to indicate that some of the
symptoms of the disorder are present even though the criteria to make
the diagnosis have not been met.

Those who have advanced the pediatric bipolar disorder diagnosis
have not followed the criteria for the diagnosis outlined in the *DSM-
IV*. Instead, many prominent psychiatric researchers have trumpeted
to the public a "disorder" that uses the same name that has long been
used to define a widely recognized illness but does not meet its *DSM-IV*
criteria. About half of all children diagnosed with bipolar disorder are
given the diagnosis "bipolar disorder NOS" (Axelson et al., 2006;
Galanter et al., 2009). As will be shown in the next chapter, the bipolar
disorder NOS diagnosis is a verbal sleight of hand that creates the illusion that a patient without bipolar disorder has the disorder. There
is no *DSM* entity for a children's version of bipolar disorder. There is

simply bipolar disorder, and all of its criteria apply irrespective of the age of the patient.

REFERENCES

American Psychiatric Association. (2000). *Diagnostic and Statistical Manual of Mental Disorders* (4th ed. Text Revision ed.). Washington, DC: American Psychiatric Association.

Axelson, D., Birmaher, B., Strober, M., Gill, M.K., Valeri, S., Chiappetta, L., et al. (2006). Phenomenology of children and adolescents with bipolar spectrum disorders. *Arch Gen Psychiatry, 63*(10), 1139–1148.

Galanter, C.A., Pagar, D.L., Oberg, P.P., Wong, C., Davies, M., & Jensen, P.S. (2009). Symptoms leading to a bipolar diagnosis: a phone survey of child and adolescent psychiatrists. *J Child Adolesc Psychopharmacol, 19*(6), 641–647.

Goodwin, F.K., & Jamison, K.R. (2007). Clinical Description. In F. K. Jamison & K.R. Jamison (Eds.), *Manic-Depressive Illness: Bipolar Disorders and Recurrent Depression* (pp. 29–87). Oxford: Oxford University Press.

Healy, D. (2009). Trussed in Evidence? Ambiguities at the Interface between Clinical Evidence and Clinical Practice. *Transcultural Psychiatry, 46*(1), 16–37.

Jamison, K. R. (2004). *Exuberance: A Passion for Life*. New York: Vintage.

Jamison, K.R. (2007). *An Unquiet Mind: A Memoir of Moods and Madness*. New York: Alfred A. Knopf.

Sadler, J.Z. (2009). The instrument metaphor, hyponarrativity, and the generic clinician. In P. James (Ed.), *Philosophical Perspectives on Technology and Psychiatry* (pp. 23–33). New York: Oxford University Press.

2

Pediatric Bipolar Disorder

The appearance of adult bipolar disorder is so dramatically different from the appearance of child bipolar disorder that it's hard to imagine how the two could be confused. Adults with bipolar disorder have clear-cut episodes of very distinctive behavior: severe overexcitement, irritability, or highs ("mania") that last for weeks followed by crushing lows or depression that also last for weeks. The adult is said to have a "cycle" or "mood swing" when moving from one episode to another. In between the highs and lows are long periods without them. In adults the episodes are recognizable by family, friends, and even the patient as being significantly different from how the patient usually behaves.

The child diagnosed with bipolar disorder, on the other hand, has chronic, almost constant symptoms that characterize, rather than deviate from, the child's usual behavior. The typical elementary school aged child diagnosed with bipolar disorder tends to be easily angered and can have several angry episodes per day in the form of screaming, tantrums, cursing, and biting. Though the anger may sometimes seem to "come from nowhere," it occurs most often when the child does not get his or her own way, is asked to do something he or she does not want to do, or is criticized or slighted in some way. Not surprisingly, the anger usually ends when the child manages to get what the child wants. Before achieving this goal, the frustrated child can yell, curse, kick, or throw things. The tendency to react to frustration by becoming enraged is constant. In serious cases the child will attack others, including classmates, parents, teachers, or principals. The potential for this kind of behavior is chronic and can flare several times a day. Many parents report feeling as though they are "walking on eggshells" around their children. As these children age, they become more difficult to control because of their increase in size and strength.

How is it possible that two such different disorders could be confused for one another? As discussed earlier, the "A" criterion for a manic episode is defined as a "distinct period of abnormally and persistently elevated, expansive, or irritable mood, lasting at least 1 week (or any duration if hospitalization is necessary)." Proponents of the diagnosis of pediatric bipolar disorder point to the chronic irritability of their patients as evidence of a manic episode. Although it is true that irritability is sufficient to meet the "A" criterion of a manic episode, it is also crucial to the diagnosis that this irritability is a *distinct period* that is different from the patient's normal functioning.

The intense anger typically found in children who have been diagnosed as having bipolar disorder is a chronic problem. These children are not in a distinct state that is different from their usual selves; they are prone to anger or irritability all the time. Often, the problem has been present for many years, and typically it continues long after the diagnosis of bipolar disorder has been made. Unlike adults with bipolar disorder, these children do not have weeks or months of apparently normal behavior. Their irritability, if not always present, is always a felt threat. So while they may meet the "A" criterion for mood—irritability—they do not meet the "A" criterion for a distinct state. This is not insignificant, as these *DSM-IV* criteria must be met in order for the diagnosis to be applicable.

One major group advocating for the diagnosis of pediatric bipolar disorder in children claims to resolve this discrepancy by recasting each angry outburst as a distinct state. In this view, the child with outbursts of anger or irritability is considered to have "cycled" with each outburst. Every minor change in mood that occurs during the ordinary course of a day is counted as a cycle. For children easily provoked to anger, there can be many such cycles per day (Geller, Tillman, & Bolhofner, 2007). Of course, these transient shifts of mood during the course of the child's day are not comparable to the cycles of actual bipolar disorder that usually occur over much longer periods—weeks to months—in adolescents and adults. Instead, the diagnosis of pediatric bipolar disorder in these irritable children is an incorrect interpretation of a frequently observed childhood behavior: temper tantrums. These outbursts are fundamentally different from the complete psychological reorganization that occurs during a bipolar disorder cycle.

PEDIATRIC BIPOLAR DISORDER
AS ADHD AND ODD

Children misdiagnosed with bipolar disorder typically do have serious difficulties that can seem similar to some of the symptoms of mania. These include irritability, distractibility, and talkativeness, among others. But these difficulties are already well known to child psychiatrists and are well described in the *DSM-IV* as the less serious (and far more treatable) diagnoses of attention deficit hyperactivity disorder (ADHD) and oppositional defiant disorder (ODD) (Carlson, 2005). Most of the *DSM-IV* symptoms of mania can easily be matched to one of these disorders. These diagnoses are more fitting still when you consider that, unlike mania, ADHD and ODD are chronic disorders. The symptoms are characteristically present most of the time and do not have to meet the bipolar disorder criterion of being different from the patient's usual self.

It is estimated that anywhere from 60% to 90% of children diagnosed with bipolar disorder are also diagnosed with ADHD (Galanter et al., 2009; Geller et al., 2000; Safer, 2009; Singh et al., 2006). ADHD is characterized by concentration difficulty and often by physical overactivity and difficulty controlling impulses. By *DSM-IV* definition, some symptoms are evident before the age of seven, and the diagnosis becomes a consideration in children having difficulty in the early elementary school years. The children may be restless and fidgety and have difficulty staying in their seats. They often have trouble paying attention, organizing themselves, and finishing their school work. ADHD is found in 7% of elementary school age children. In general, it is diagnosed in boys two times more often than girls and is the most common disorder treated in child psychiatry clinics. The *DSM-IV* criteria for the diagnosis are listed in Table 2.1.

From the perspective of a child psychiatrist, the case of Nathaniel illustrates some of the typical features of ADHD. Nathaniel is a nine-year-old who has always had difficulty remaining in his seat in class. Now in third grade, he frequently leaves his seat to talk to other children and to engage in activities unrelated to the lesson being taught. Even when Nathaniel is in his seat, he is in motion. He drums with his hands and taps his feet. The teacher reports that he is unable to attend to lessons and is in danger of having to repeat the year despite his obviously high intelligence. Often, he fails to bring his homework assignments home, requires his parents' help to complete the assignments when he does bring them home, and then frequently neglects to bring the completed assignments back to school. On those rare occa-

TABLE 2.1. DSM-IV Diagnostic Criteria for Attention Deficit/ Hyperactivity Disorder

A. Either (1) or (2)

  (1) six (or more) of the following symptoms of inattention have persisted for at least 6 months to a degree that is maladaptive and inconsistent with developmental level:

  Inattention
  (a) often fails to give close attention to details or makes careless mistakes in schoolwork, work, or other activities
  (b) often has difficulty sustaining attention in tasks or play activities
  (c) often does not seem to listen when spoken to directly
  (d) often does not follow through on instructions and fails to finish schoolwork, chores, or duties in the workplace (not due to oppositional behavior or failure to understand instructions)
  (e) often has difficulty organizing tasks and activities
  (f) often avoids, dislikes, or is reluctant to engage in tasks that require sustained mental effort (such as schoolwork or homework)
  (g) often loses things necessary for tasks or activities (e.g., toys, school assignments, pencils, books, or tools)
  (h) is often easily distracted by extraneous stimuli
  (i) is often forgetful in daily activities

  (2) six (or more) of the following symptoms of hyperactivity-impulsivity have persisted for at least 6 months to a degree that is maladaptive and inconsistent with developmental level:

  Hyperactivity/Impulsivity
  Hyperactivity
  (a) often fidgets with hands or feet or squirms in seat
  (b) often leaves seat in classroom or in other situations in which remaining seated is expected
  (c) often runs about or climbs excessively in situations in which it is inappropriate (in adolescents or adults, may be limited to subjective feelings of restlessness)
  (d) often has difficulty playing or engaging in leisure activities quietly
  (e) is often "on the go" or often acts as if "driven by a motor"
  (f) often talks excessively

  Impulsivity
  (g) often blurts out answers before questions have been completed
  (h) often has difficulty awaiting turn
  (i) often interrupts or intrudes on others (e.g., butts into conversations or games)

B. Some hyperactive-impulsive or inattentive symptoms that caused impairment were present before age 7 years.

C. Some impairment from the symptoms is present in two or more settings (e.g., at school [or work] and at home).

D. There must be clear evidence of clinically significant impairment in social, academic, or occupational functioning.

**TABLE 2.1. DSM-IV Diagnostic Criteria for Attention Deficit/
Hyperactivity Disorder (*Continued*)**

E. The symptoms do not occur exclusively during the course of a Pervasive
Developmental Disorder, Schizophrenia, or other Psychotic Disorder and
are not better accounted for by another mental disorder (e.g., Mood Disorder, Anxiety Disorder, or a Personality Disorder).

(Reprinted with permission from the *Diagnostic and Statistical Manual of Mental Disorders,
Fourth Edition,* Text Revision [Copyright 2000]. American Psychiatric Association.)

sions when he does complete the assignment at home and return it to
school, he often neglects to hand it in to the teacher.

At home, Nathaniel often seems as if he's disobeying his parents. For
example, if they ask him to clean up his bedroom, they may find that a
half an hour later he's playing with some toys in the bedroom but his
clothes remain scattered on the floor. When asked about his failure to
clean up his room as they requested, he explains that he "forgot" what
they asked him to do. At dinner, Nathaniel prefers to eat standing up
in the dining room and frequently runs to the TV room to glimpse the
cartoon he had been watching before dinner began. Despite his distractibility, Nathaniel loves to play computer games, and his parents report
that he can pay attention to something as long as he's interested in it. If
he is not interested, which is frequent, he can't pay attention. Because of
his constant talking he is regarded by the family as a "motor mouth."
According to the parents, this behavior had been going on at home and
at school since Nathaniel was five years old.

The ADHD diagnosis easily includes many of the behaviors described in the misdiagnosis of childhood bipolar disorder. Both the
bipolar disorder child and the ADHD child are described as being excessively talkative. In general, people who talk fast also have rapid
thoughts. Clinically it is common for children with ADHD to admit
to racing thoughts, which is likewise the case for the bipolar disorder
child. Both are also described as being easily distracted. The "increase
in goal directed activity" of the child with bipolar disorder is similar to
the ADHD symptom "is often on the go or often acts as if driven by a
motor." ADHD patients have a strong need to be "busy." The item refers
primarily to motor activity in ADHD children, but the need to be doing
things could be included in that item. Adults with ADHD have a difficult time with beach vacations because lying on a beach doing nothing is
very hard for many of them. The mania symptom, "decreased need for
sleep," is also reported often by parents, who explain that their ADHD

children were always poor sleepers who would rock their cribs, wander the house at night, and now seem to require less sleep than their non-ADHD siblings. Table 2.2 outlines these similarities, along with the corresponding references to the *DSM-IV* diagnoses for these disorders (see Table 2.2).

Although the ADHD diagnosis does account for several of the symptoms of mania, it does not account for the angry behaviors that typify children diagnosed with bipolar disorder. Anger, irritability, and aggression are not *DSM* symptoms of ADHD. Within the universe of ADHD children, however, there is a sizeable group who are very angry and irritable. When this irritability is added to the ADHD symptoms, the child is indistinguishable from the child diagnosed with bipolar disorder. My contention is that irritable children with ADHD are not childhood bipolar disorder patients at all; rather they are ADHD patients who are angry and irritable.

Irritability is a symptom that is found frequently in many psychiatric disorders (Safer, 2009). It is a crucial feature of oppositional defiant disorder (ODD), an extremely common psychiatric disorder of childhood that is closely associated with, and often accompanied by, ADHD. Oppositional defiant disorder is a *DSM-IV* diagnosis that specifies a number of the most important problems found in children misdiagnosed with bipolar disorder. Children with ODD are quick to defy adult request or demands and often refuse to do what they are asked to do. The criteria for diagnosing the disorder include often losing one's temper,

TABLE 2.2. Comparison of Selected DSM-IV Mania and ADHD Symptoms

Mania Symptoms	ADHD Symptoms
(B.3.) more talkative than usual or pressure to keep talking	(2 f) often talks excessively (2 g) often blurts out answers before questions have been completed (2 i) often interrupts or intrudes on others (e.g., butts into conversations or games)
(B.4.) flight of ideas or subjective experience that thoughts are racing	(2 f) often talks excessively
(B.5.) distractibility (i.e., attention too easily drawn to unimportant or irrelevant external stimuli)	(1 h) is often easily distracted by extraneous stimuli
(B.6.) increase in goal-directed activity (either socially, at work or school, or sexually) or psychomotor agitation	(2 e) is often "on the go" or often acts as if "driven by a motor"

often arguing with adults, and often feeling angry and resentful (see Table 2.3). These children frequently exhibit behavioral problems in school. They refuse to follow school rules and standard social conventions. They may be suspended, expelled and transferred to special education settings. Aggression in childhood is not tolerated by institutions charged with caring for children. It quickly leads to educational placements outside of regular education classrooms and begins a journey of stigmatization that puts the aggressive child at an important disadvantage compared to the child's nonaggressive peers.

I work as a consultant to a special education school, and it is not unusual to encounter at least a few 7- to 12-year-old children with combined ADHD and ODD in the hallways outside of the classroom during class time. Their behaviors exemplify the ODD diagnosis. These children have defiantly left the class, refusing to return. They are found kicking lockers, cursing at adults who attempt to intervene, and in general making every effort to disobey and disrupt school routines. When they are in class, they are often impulsive, restless, rude, loud, threatening, and defiant.

The diagnosis of ODD is easy to recognize, and the *DSM-IV* criteria are self-explanatory. The recommended treatment for ODD is behavior

---

TABLE 2.3. DSM-IV Diagnostic Criteria for Oppositional Defiant Disorder

---

A. A pattern of negativistic, hostile, and defiant behavior lasting at least 6 months, during which four(or more) of the following are present:
    (1) often loses temper
    (2) often argues with adults
    (3) often actively defies or refuses to comply with adults' request or rules
    (4) often deliberately annoys people
    (5) often blames others for his or her mistakes or misbehavior
    (6) is often touchy or easily annoyed by others
    (7) is often angry and resentful
    (8) is often spiteful or vindictive
    Note: Consider a criterion met only if the behavior occurs more frequently than is typically observed in individuals of comparable age and developmental level.
B. The disturbance in behavior causes clinically significant impairment in social, academic or occupational functioning.
C. The behaviors do not occur exclusively during the course of a Psychotic or Mood Disorder.
D. Criteria are not met for Conduct Disorder, and, if the individual is age 18 years or older, criteria are not met for Antisocial Personality Disorder.

(Reprinted with permission from the *Diagnostic and Statistical Manual of Mental Disorders, Fourth Edition*, Text Revision [Copyright 2000]. American Psychiatric Association.)

modification, sometimes in combination with medication. ODD often seems to account for the aggressive behavior in children that leads to the incorrect diagnosis of pediatric bipolar disorder.

This was the case for Lucy, a girl diagnosed with bipolar disorder whose symptoms clearly indicated the presence of ADHD and ODD. Lucy was a 12-year-old girl with eight previous child psychiatric hospitalizations. I saw her as a consultant on an inpatient unit during her ninth hospitalization. She had recently been expelled from a special education setting for severely misbehaving children after she had been in the program for less than one week. She was then placed in a day hospital program but only lasted there for two days as her frequent and severe aggression required readmission to the hospital.

Lucy had a long-standing history of violence. Her symptoms included constant refusal to conform to rules, cursing, physical aggression against teachers, throwing chairs, and biting peers. She repeatedly ran out of classrooms and she ran away from home on a weekly basis. Lucy's anger, defiance, and temper tantrums were first noted at age three. At that time she was also noted to be restless, overactive, and talkative, which continued throughout her childhood and was clearly evident during the interview. As a young child, Lucy was placed in a special education preschool program for emotionally disturbed children. She cursed frequently in the classroom and challenged her teachers constantly by not following classroom routines. She was diagnosed with bipolar disorder at the age of five and had been treated since then with a number of medications used for adult bipolar disorder. Despite these medications, her many hospitalizations, and an array of special education and mental health services, she did not respond to treatment.

When I interviewed Lucy during her most recent hospitalization, she reported that she *could* sit still and pay attention but that she intentionally chose not to. Although she very clearly met the criteria for ADHD, she seemed to need to maintain the illusion for herself that she had control over her behavior. ADHD had not been considered as a diagnosis, and she had never been treated with medication for it.

This case illustrates many of the aspects of behavior that lead to the misdiagnosis of child bipolar disorder. The most conspicuous feature of this case, and of most children who receive the diagnosis, is excessive irritability and anger. The symptoms of ODD dominate the appearance of the so-called childhood bipolar disorder patient. Most of the *DSM-IV* symptoms of mania can also easily be matched to those of ADHD and ODD. There doesn't seem to be much difference between combined ODD and ADHD and the description of the child bipolar disorder patient. The clinical reality is that there is no difference.

My view of pediatric bipolar disorder is that it is almost always severe oppositional defiant disorder combined with severe ADHD. These two *DSM-IV* diagnoses account for all of the observed "bipolar" symptoms. Also, both ADHD and ODD are relatively common diagnoses for elementary school aged children. The co-occurrence of these two disorders is frequently encountered as well, in contrast to the rarity of an actual case of bipolar disorder in childhood. The combined diagnosis of ADHD and ODD is the best and most likely explanation for the anger found in these elementary school age children. There is no need to add the additional diagnosis of bipolar disorder; it is confusing and misleading to do so.

There are three critical reasons for redefining most cases of child bipolar disorder as ADHD and ODD.

First, and most important, ADHD and ODD are the diagnoses these children seem to have; together they provide a better measure of the children's actual difficulties than does the diagnosis of bipolar disorder. The symptoms of ADHD and ODD are characteristically present most of the time and do not have to meet the bipolar disorder criterion of being distinctly different from the patient's usual self. ADHD symptoms, in particular, must appear early in the child's life and persist over time. By *DSM-IV* definition, they are stable and must have been present since before the age of seven. In contrast, the *DSM-IV* symptoms of mania must represent a change from usual behavior—that is, to count as mania, an increase or decrease in symptoms must occur with the change in mood. Most advocates for the childhood bipolar disorder diagnosis ignore this requirement. Yet it is a major violation of *DSM-IV* to label what are essentially long-standing symptoms of ADHD or ODD as transitory symptoms of bipolar disorder.

Second, ADHD and ODD are relatively easy to treat compared to bipolar disorder. Bipolar disorder can be treated in adults, but often it is difficult. Lithium, the most effective treatment known, only works in 50% of adult patients. Antiseizure medications, also used in adults, have not been researched sufficiently for use in the treatment of pediatric bipolar disorder patients. What little is known is not encouraging; there is little evidence that they work in children. Antipsychotic medications are used increasingly in bipolar disorder children, and some have very recently been FDA approved in the 10–17-year-old age range. Yet these have an array of side effects that many parents and children find unacceptable.

In contrast to the lack of understanding of the treatment of child bipolar disorder, the treatment of ADHD is very well understood. It is effective and safe. Many hundreds of studies on the treatment of the disorder with stimulant medications have been conducted since the

1930s, and they have demonstrated that these medications are an effective treatment for the disorder. One of the most stern clinical rules in medicine is that it is vital not to fail to recognize and diagnose a treatable condition. In Lucy's case, as in a number of cases of childhood bipolar disorder, ADHD was missed as a diagnosis; often it is not treated even when it is identified. Effective treatment of ADHD often resolves many of the symptoms that led to the child's diagnosis of bipolar disorder. As a clinician, I am always interested in redefining a problem that is untreatable into a problem that is treatable.

Third, an older tradition in child psychiatry suggests that when there is ambiguity about a diagnosis, a less serious diagnosis is preferable to a more malignant diagnosis. With time, the clinical situation might become more clear and the malignant diagnosis might indeed have not been selected. In the interim, the child and family would not have been burdened with the anxiety and the more hazardous treatments of the more serious diagnosis.

THE DEVELOPMENT OF THE DIAGNOSIS OF PEDIATRIC BIPOLAR DISORDER

For many years the general view among child psychiatrists was that aggressive, hyperactive school age children usually had ADHD and often had ODD as well. Sometime around the middle part of the 1990s this view began to change. At that time, two distinguished child psychiatrists, Joseph Biederman, MD, at Harvard University, and Barbara Geller, MD, at Washington University, independently began to report that there was something more than ADHD and ODD that was troubling severely disruptive school age children and adolescents. The additional crucial diagnosis that had been overlooked, according to Drs. Geller and Biederman, was bipolar disorder. They went on to define pediatric bipolar disorder for child psychiatrists, creating a large amount of excitement in the profession and in the public. Working independently, they and their colleagues continue to study and write frequent articles about the disorder.

It is significant that these two prominent research groups differ in their descriptions and criteria for the diagnosis. Dr. Biederman and his colleagues argue that pediatric bipolar disorder is defined by severe aggression; Dr. Geller and her colleagues argue that pediatric bipolar disorder is defined by grandiosity and elation. That two of the leading child psychiatric investigators of this area could not agree on the fundamentals of the clinical appearance of these children does nothing to allay misgivings about the accuracy of this novel diagnosis. The difficulty in pinpointing exactly what characterizes pediatric bipolar disorder is one of the crucial issues in the controversy surrounding the diagnosis. It will be useful for our purposes, therefore, to understand exactly how these independent conclusions were drawn.

Dr. Biederman, who is credited with introducing the contemporary concept of pediatric bipolar disorder to the child psychiatric community, is a full professor of psychiatry at Harvard. Prior to introducing this new diagnosis he had published a large number of careful studies of ADHD as well as studies of other child psychiatric disorders. He has received many grants from NIMH and works closely advising and performing studies for the pharmaceutical industry. He is tireless in his efforts to make child psychiatry more scientific by the use of carefully performed research studies. He is a charismatic public speaker, and his influence in the field is of child psychiatry cannot be exaggerated.

Dr. Biederman and his colleagues (including distinguished child psychiatric researchers Timothy Wilens, MD, Janet Wozniak, MD, and Stephen Faraone, PhD), published numerous studies of pediatric bipolar disorder in rapid succession in the mid- to late 1990s, as noted by Geller (Geller, 1997). The first study, which served as a model for many of the subsequent studies, evaluated all 262 children aged 12 years and younger who had been referred to the Pediatric Psychopharmacology Unit of the Child Psychiatry Service at Massachusetts General Hospital for evaluation and treatment. The data collection began in 1991, but the authors do not provide an end date. The children had not been referred because of a particular diagnosis but simply for evaluation and possible treatment with medication. Each child received an evaluation that consisted of a clinical interview of the parent about the child and a psychiatric research interview of the parent about the child. The psychiatric research interview assessed symptoms for all psychiatric disorders. The children themselves were not interviewed.

Of the 262 children who had been referred for evaluation and treatment, 43 (16%) were declared by the authors to have mania. Forty-two of the 43 manic children (98%) also had ADHD. More than three-fourths of the children who met the criteria for mania (77%) did so because of extreme and persistent irritability (33 of the 43). These manic patients were notable, in particular, for their marked levels of aggression. The young age of mania onset was dramatic as well. The authors report the age of onset of the mania in 70% of the manic subjects to have been before the age of five. At that time the diagnosis of mania in a child that young was very rare (Wozniak et al., 1995). Although the authors used a number of careful research procedures in an effort to reach an accurate diagnosis, incredibly, they did not interview the child patients. Instead, information about the children's behavior was gathered in interviews with their parents. In clinical work, it is legally required that the patient be seen during a patient evaluation. I doubt that there is a managed care company in the country that would pay for a child psychiatric evaluation in which the patient was not seen. It is also a traditional part of medical culture for the doctor always to see the patient. It becomes habitual during long nights of providing care during internships and years of post-graduate medical education. It is a source of specific professional pride for child psychiatrists that they can gain meaningful information from interviewing child patients. It is not uncommon for the physician or diagnostician to see a patient quite differently from how the patient has been described by the parent. In a research study purporting to describe a new diagnosis, it is hard to imagine relying solely on parent reporting and not interviewing the patients.

In the discussion section of the article, the authors noted that the children seemed to have a level of aggression that qualified them for a diagnosis of mania, and the authors laid down the challenge for the child psychiatric field to recognize these aggressive children as having early bipolar disorder, based on the severity of their aggression. In later articles, the Biederman group continued the position that aggressive severity differentiated pediatric bipolar disorder from ADHD (Biederman, 1995; Biederman et al., 1999; Faraone et al., 1997; Wozniak & Biederman, 1996). Bipolar disorder, however, is an entirely different type of disorder. According to the *DSM-IV*, ADHD is classified as a "Disruptive Behavior Disorder" while bipolar disorder is an "Affective [mood] Disorder"—a completely different category. The Biederman group mistakenly treats what is only a difference in severity as a major difference in type of disorder. *DSM-IV* bipolar disorder is not on a continuum with ADHD or ADHD plus ODD, as these studies incorrectly suggested. Aside from the issue of severity of aggressive symptoms, which is insufficient for confirming a *DSM-IV* diagnosis of mania, Biederman's group failed to provide any persuasive evidence that the children had bipolar disorder.

In a related study (Biederman et al., 1995), Biederman and his group again did not interview the child patients (Biederman et al., 1995). In this new study, the authors had the same group of parents mentioned above complete a symptom checklist, called the Child Behavior Checklist (CBCL), to determine whether or not the children's scores corresponded to the diagnosis of mania that had been made in the first study. Not surprisingly, as that initial diagnosis was based exclusively on parent reporting, they did correspond. The authors conclude that the CBCL questionnaire can be used to diagnose bipolar disorder. Although the CBCL was designed to analyze a child's emotional and behavioral health, it is not intended to assess for mania or bipolar disorder. Investigators who study bipolar disorder in children, however, continue to use it (Biederman et al., 2009; Luby & Belden, 2006).

The studies of the 262 children, of course, do not tell us whether any of the children actually had bipolar disorder. The studies merely confirm that the parents told an interviewer in the first study approximately the same material about their children that they wrote on a paper-and-pencil questionnaire in the second study. The children in these two studies were not interviewed, and Biederman's group failed to provide any other persuasive evidence that the children had bipolar disorder. Perhaps because of the enormous amount of influence Dr. Biederman and his group have in the field, many child psychiatrists nonetheless adopted his views on the existence of the disorder following the publication of these and similar studies.

Barbara Geller, MD, began to write and speak about pediatric bipolar disorder at about the same time Dr. Biederman began to present his work. She is well known in child psychiatry as a distinguished academic psychiatrist who recently retired from the prestigious Washington University of St. Louis. She has received numerous grants from NIMH and has published prolifically on bipolar disorder in children. She, too, is a strong and major influence on contemporary child psychiatric views of pediatric bipolar disorder.

Dr. Geller has criticized the pediatric bipolar disorder work of Dr. Biederman and his colleagues on similar grounds to the criticisms made here. She highlights the fact that there were no interviews of children. She also makes the point that irritability is a frequently encountered symptom found in many different diagnoses and thus cannot be helpful in making the specific diagnosis of bipolar disorder.

Nonetheless, Dr. Geller and colleagues continued to support the validity of the diagnosis. Initially, she and her colleagues believed that children with bipolar disorder had several symptoms of mania beyond what are found in aggressive children with ADHD and ODD. Eventually they settled on two: grandiosity and elation. Whether they appeared independently or combined, these two symptoms were seen by Dr. Geller as the "cardinal symptoms" of pediatric bipolar disorder. "Cardinal" is not a *DSM-IV* term. It is not in the index of the *DSM-IV* and is not part of day-to-day mental health jargon. Dr. Geller defines a "cardinal symptom" as one that is unique to a diagnosis in *DSM-IV* terms (Geller et al., 2004). Grandiosity, however, which is an over-inflated sense of self-worth or self-importance, is found in a number of *DSM-IV* diagnoses. Narcissistic personality disorder, for example, refers to a condition in which patients have an excessive self-regard, sense of entitlement, and belief that others are inferior. Grandiosity is found in normal child development as well. It is not unique to mania and therefore is not a cardinal symptom by Dr. Geller's own definition (Wozniak et al., 2005).

The case of Alexis demonstrates some of the misconceptions about grandiosity and how it is sometimes misinterpreted as diagnostic of pediatric bipolar disorder.

Alexis was an 11-year-old girl who attended a private school for troubled children. She had been diagnosed with bipolar disorder at a center for the study of child bipolar disorder and had been placed on a variety of mood-stabilizing agents, including lithium, valproic acid, and carbamazepine. The medications had been initiated about two years previously, which roughly coincided with her admission to the school. The medications were not working. During her two years at the school she performed poorly and had not demonstrated academic or clinical improvement. Her parents had requested a private psychiatric consultation. When I first met Alexis, she had been refusing to attend class or do any work for many months. Her failure to participate in the classroom or in any other school activity led the school to decide to terminate her enrollment in two months at the end of the school year.

Alexis came from a high-achieving, upper-social-class family. Her parents and close relatives served on the boards of her city's largest corporations. The family's power and affluence lent a larger-than-life quality to much of what they did. For the most part Alexis refused to talk with me during our sessions, which made it difficult to develop a coherent understanding of her current problems. Information gathered from the parents and other relatives was also of little help in clarifying the diagnosis. Alexis was a talented artist and spent her sessions with me drawing very elaborate Renaissance-like drawings of people in a large leather-bound book. She was also a child actor in an adult Shakespearean theatrical group in the city and spent long hours at play rehearsals. The family felt that she was talented and highly intelligent but was bored by schoolwork and by the activities of children her own age.

During Alexis's early elementary school years, doctors and other professionals had suggested that she might have ADHD because of her difficulties concentrating on schoolwork. Her parents disagreed with these diagnostic impressions because of the mistaken belief that their daughter's many talents were inconsistent with ADHD.

In school, the teachers reported that Alexis did not do her work. She seemed unable to concentrate on it. This was less than clear, however, because she rarely made any effort in class. Her main activity during the day was to leave class and go to the teachers' lounge. Here, she tried to engage in conversations with the teachers. She preferred the teachers to the other children and had no friends at the school.

I consulted with some of the doctors who had treated her in the past. Although they felt unsure about the diagnosis of bipolar disorder, they had nevertheless treated her for it with mood stabilizers. She had been seen for several years and had had placements in a day treatment program for bipolar disorder. Though she did not respond to the treatment, she was still given the diagnosis, and the family believed the diagnosis was correct.

Clinically, Alexis's apparently arrogant refusal to participate in class work, her preference for socializing with teachers over classmates, and her preoccupation with art and Shakespearean acting suggested an element of grandiosity possibly consistent with bipolar disorder. No other symptoms of bipolar disorder, however, were present. Alexis did not have mood swings, had never had a clear-cut episode of depression or mania, had never had a week-long period of elated mood or irritability, and had no symptoms of bipolar disorder other than the possible grandiosity, which was chronic rather than episodic.

Consistent with the diagnosis of ADHD was the suggestion that her refusal to do schoolwork may have reflected difficulties in concentrating that she tried to disguise by feigning a lack of interest. Another behavior that suggested ADHD was her walking out of class, which could have reflected a symptom of overactivity. An urge to move is often concealed by leaving class to get a drink of water, go to the bathroom, or in her case, visit the teachers' lounge. Finally, the doctors who saw her in her early childhood believed she had ADHD.

Faced with certain expulsion from school, a trial of stimulant medication seemed warranted in an effort to forestall this undesirable outcome. Her mood stabilizers were stopped, and she was placed on a moderate dose of a stimulant medication. Her behavior changed immediately and dramatically. Within two or three days of starting the stimulant, she began attending classes regularly and began to work in class. The school decided to re-enroll her for the fall semester.

From a technical perspective, the response to stimulant medication alone does not confirm the diagnosis of ADHD. Performance is improved for almost everyone on stimulant medication. To merit the diagnosis of ADHD, she would have to meet other criteria for the disorder. With careful probing, it became clear that these criteria were met.

This is a good example of the not-uncommon situation in which a family avoids the diagnosis of ADHD but willingly accepts the more serious diagnosis of bipolar disorder. An inclination to be disdainful of those with ADHD and to associate bipolar disorder with the more creative interests of their daughter may have contributed to missing the ADHD diagnosis.

Alexis's case provides some information about the fate of children incorrectly diagnosed as having bipolar disorder. Had she not been diagnosed and treated for her ADHD, Alexis's problems would likely have remained intractable. For this affluent family, more expensive private boarding school for the educationally disabled would have been the next intervention. Without the correct diagnosis and treatment Alexis's pattern of failure would have continued. A persistent pattern of academic and personal failure is the fate of many children with untreated ADHD who have been diagnosed incorrectly as having bipolar disorder.

Although grandiosity is not a *DSM-IV* symptom of ODD, it is nonetheless common in patients with ODD. For example, I once had a session with a nine-year-old boy, Andrew, who had been diagnosed with ADHD and ODD and was brought in for evaluation of his severe disruptive behavior. It quickly became clear that prior to the visit Andrew had extracted an agreement from his mother that he would decide upon the medication and its dose because he knew best. When I tried to discuss various medication options, he became enraged at his mother and insisted that she abide by her promise to him. The mother acceded to his wishes and demanded that the child, rather than the child psychiatrist, decide upon the medication and dose. Andrew was grandiose in his belief that he knew more and was more powerful than his doctor. He had coerced his mother and tried to coerce me into getting his way. This mother always acceded to his wishes, and this served to confirm his distorted belief in his own power, making it virtually impossible for those outside of the home to control his behavior. This form of grandiosity is common in ODD children. As this case suggests, any challenge to authority by an oppositional child involves some degree of grandiosity.

Andrew's belief that he could refuse the demands of his powerful protectors and providers and exercise his own will required at least some overestimation of his own power. The same could be said of children who refuse to go to bed at assigned times, refuse to do homework, or refuse to comply with household rules. Any of these situations suggests that these children believe that they have the power to extract what they want from unwilling providers. Insofar as this belief is true, the need for parent counseling or family therapy to toughen parent limit-setting ability seems clear. Insofar as this belief is false, there is an element of grandiosity at play in these children's minds. Of course, in the real world there is usually a mixture of overindulgent parents combined with elements of grandiosity in the children. A parent's difficulty in setting limits on a child tends to reinforce the child's grandiosity and perception of power in the family.

The role of grandiosity in the psychology of the everyday life of the child may not be well understood. Grandiosity, expressed in the form of ambition, could play a critical role in normal child development. Geller felt that a child with no musical talent who persisted in practicing a musical instrument and had aspirations for a great musical career could be considered grandiose. It certainly seems possible, however, perhaps even likely, that such a child would find, over time, that he or she was not suited for such a career and would go on to other things. This type of grandiosity is inextricably linked to normal ambition in early adulthood as well. The belief that one can become a successful artist, excel at a sport, have a great love, or raise a child may entail some grandiosity. A modest amount of grandiosity, at least, may even be necessary for success in the world. Given these considerations, grandiosity does not seem to be a cardinal symptom of bipolar disorder because it is found in many other *DSM* disorders as well as in nonpathological situations in everyday life.

Geller's second "cardinal symptom," elated mood, is not necessarily abnormal. Elation means extreme happiness. Geller notes that the emotion is found in normal children on holidays such as birthdays or Christmas, at amusement parks, and during other joyous times of childhood. It is when this intense happiness occurs without reason or far beyond what would be expected for the circumstances that it becomes a potential psychiatric symptom. Geller and colleagues describe the elation as brief periods of silliness and giggling (Geller et al., 2002). Silliness and giggling, however, are a normal part of childhood and can be engaged in by children for a variety of reasons unrelated to bipolar disorder. Precise criteria for diagnosing pleasant mood feelings as abnormal are difficult to establish. It seems unlikely that the giggling and silliness described by these authors would be easily recognized as pathological elated mood; furthermore, the fact that the periods are brief counters characterizing them as constituting the elation of bipolar disorder, as this elation needs to last seven days or longer in *DSM-IV* to count as an episode of mania.

In adult mania, a great deal of scholarly psychiatric study has been devoted to the subject of episode length (time the symptoms are present) and cycle length (time from beginning of one episode to beginning of next), and there is considerable precedent in using these words according to the agreed-upon definitions. On several occasions Geller and her colleagues have recommended a major redefinition of these concepts in order to reflect their observations of children they have diagnosed as having pediatric bipolar disorder. They believe pediatric bipolar disorder patients switch moods more often than adult bipolar disorder patients. The shortest episode length in adult bipolar disorder is the rapid cycler who has about four cycles per year. An exceptionally rare set of adult patients with an extremely high number of cycles a year has also been described. Rather than being exceptionally rare, Geller and colleagues believe it is common for pediatric bipolar disorder patients to be "ultrarapid cyclers" (with 5–364 cycles per year) or even "ultraradian cyclers" (with more than 365 cycles a year) (Geller, Tillman, & Bolhofner, 2007; Tillman & Geller, 2003).

The contrast between adult patients having cycles lasting six months to several years and child patients having numerous cycles throughout a day is striking. It is obviously a mistake to identify these very different phenomena as the same.

Parents of patients often come to believe that every temporary shift in mood is a "mood swing" or "cycle" and anxiously point to a childish pout or temper tantrum as evidence that their child has bipolar disorder. During an evaluation session a parent may point to a grumpy child and announce, "See? It's starting again. He's having another mood swing." Geller's concept of ultraradian cycles lends credibility to this obvious parental misinterpretation. These "mood swings" or "cycles" are entirely different from those seen in *DSM-IV* bipolar disorder.

A recent publication by several NIMH psychiatrists stated unambiguously that *DSM-IV* criteria had to be met in order to diagnose bipolar disorder in children and adolescents (Leibenluft et al., 2003). The paper strongly underscored the necessity of episodic behaviors in which *all* of the child's behaviors changed depending upon the change in the mood of the child, as *DSM-IV* requires. All mood swings, even the briefest, require that there is a shift of the patient's B group of *DSM-IV* symptoms such as elation, distractibility, grandiosity, etc. The mood and the behaviors cannot be the usual mood and behaviors the child displays. The child has to be different from his or her usual self. The NIMH group is confident that such patients exist during adolescence but seems uncertain that prepubertal children could actually meet the *DSM-IV* criteria for episodes. Rapid mood shifts in children, such as those described above, do not include changes in these other symptoms and therefore cannot count toward a diagnosis of bipolar disorder.

BIPOLAR DISORDER IN THE VERY YOUNG

The risks, failures of judgment, and bad science of pediatric bipolar disorder are even more apparent in preschool children than they are in elementary school age children. There is more of a divorce from

DSM-IV criteria, and the risks of medication may be greater because of the preschool child's lower weight and physical immaturity. The potential for diagnostic error is also greater; there is a greater chance of incorrectly deciding that behavioral issues are due to a serious psychiatric disorder rather than due to simple developmental, psychological, or family problems. It is widely appreciated that preschoolers are more sensitive than are older children to fluctuations in family functioning, which can result in a variety of troublesome behaviors.

Preschool children are less well studied than older children in psychiatry. There are less medication studies in these age groups and less clinical prescribing experience. The leading scholar of bipolar disorder in preschool children is Joan Luby, MD, of Washington University. A colleague of Dr. Geller, Dr. Luby has published several important studies on bipolar disorder in preschool children.

In an elaborate and careful NIMH-funded study, Dr. Luby had the parents of 305 preschool children interviewed by trained raters using an interview specifically designed to study depression and mania in preschool children (Luby & Belden, 2006). The children themselves were not interviewed. Based on the parental interviews, 21 of the preschool children were diagnosed as having bipolar disorder, and all of these children had depression as well. Fifty-four additional children had depression without bipolar disorder. The children diagnosed with both bipolar disorder and depression had more severe depression than the children diagnosed with depression without bipolar disorder. It has been my experience that these subtle distinctions are difficult enough to make in adults with a cooperative adult patient speaking directly to a psychiatrist. It strains credibility to believe they can be made accurately in preschoolers without ever having seen the child.

In another study based largely on the same group of patients, Dr. Luby reported that preschool children with grandiosity, elation, and hypersexuality (precocious interest in sex and sexual behaviors) were likely to have bipolar disorder (Luby & Belden, 2008). Again, the existence of these symptoms is based solely on parent reports, which are surely open to alternative interpretations than the children having bipolar disorder. It also seems unlikely that the parents were capable of evaluating symptoms such as grandiosity and elation in their preschool children. Most child psychiatrists, including myself, would be challenged when asked to weigh the significance of elation, grandiosity, and hypersexuality behaviors in an evaluation of a preschool child that they were actually observing. Asking parents of preschool children to report on these behaviors in the absence of some confirmatory professional observation of the child makes the assessment incomplete. This is especially significant because Dr. Luby asks the reader to believe in an entirely new disorder that has not been previously described in the psychiatric literature.

As was mentioned in discussion of Dr. Biederman's studies of mania in childhood, it is common knowledge that children must be seen in order to be evaluated. Dr. Luby acknowledges the failure to evaluate the children as a limitation of her study yet nonetheless seems confident in her findings. Absent some direct observation of the child, however, it is difficult to be persuaded that these preschool children actually had bipolar disorder.

Dr. Biederman's group also reported a study of 165 preschool children aged four years to six years who were diagnosed with ADHD. Of these preschool children, 26%, or 42, were also diagnosed as having bipolar disorder. This group of children was compared with an older group of 381 children aged seven to nine years who were diagnosed with ADHD. Of these older children, 69 (18%) were also diagnosed with bipolar disorder (Wilens et al., 2002). In general, these are high rates of bipolar disorder. The Biederman group also reported that the preschoolers had an average onset of their bipolar disorder at about two and a half years of age and the school age children at three years, seven months. The authors warn that reluctance to treat bipolar disorder children in their preschool years will lead to disturbed children in the future.

These types of cautions about the consequences of failing to treat the disorder at younger and younger ages are undoubtedly contributing to the dramatic increases in the diagnoses of the disorder in these age groups. As a consequence of these dire warnings, more children (and younger children) are exposed to the risk of misdiagnoses and treatment with potentially dangerous medications to little purpose.

A different view of psychopathology in the preschool years is offered by Drs. Speltz, McClellan, and colleagues. They studied 92 boys age four years to five years, five months, whom they believed were similar to the preschool group studied by the Biederman group. All of the children had ODD and about half also had ADHD. The Speltz and McClellan group followed their preschoolers for two years and, unlike the Biederman group, did not find a single case of bipolar disorder at the beginning or end of their study (Speltz et al., 1999).

The difference in the results of the two studies produced a fascinating exchange of letters between the two research groups. The Speltz group expressed the concern that the study of the Biederman group would contribute to the overdiagnosis of bipolar disorder (McClellan & Speltz, 2003). The Biederman group stood by their results and made a comment that is especially relevant to this book: "We find perplexing the notion of Drs. McClellan and Speltz that publishing data in peer-reviewed journals on a particular subject leads to an epidemic of diagnosis in children. Since when does awareness cause a disorder?" (Wilens et al., 2003, p. 129). The Biederman group seemed to minimize the powerful effect of the combination of the persuasiveness of a scientific finding with the prestige of Harvard University and the exceptional influence of this particular group of investigators on the field of child psychiatry.

Another useful corrective to the preschooler studies of Luby and Biederman is a recent published work of Birmaher and colleagues (2010). Dr. Birmaher is a longtime investigator of pediatric bipolar disorder and the recipient of numerous NIMH grants on the disorder. He is regarded as a careful, thoughtful, and highly capable researcher and one who regularly diagnoses pediatric bipolar disorder in his research studies. He studied 121 two- to five-year-old children in families in which one parent had bipolar disorder and 102 two- to five-year-old children in families in which neither parent had bipolar disorder. The interviewers of the children did not know if the parents had bipolar disorder. None of the preschool children from the bipolar disorder parent group had a bipolar I disorder diagnosis. This runs counter to what many pediatric bipolar disorder proponents would have predicted.

ONE AUTHORITATIVE VIEW

Dr. Gabrielle Carlson, MD, a professor of psychiatry and pediatrics and director of the division of child and adolescent psychiatry at State University of New York at Stony Brook, has been investigating bipolar disorder in children and adolescents for decades. She has authored numerous studies and articles about the disorder and serves almost as an unofficial referee regarding the diagnosis. She regularly chairs national conferences about research on the disorder. She recently authored the pediatric bipolar disorder sections in the authoritative Goodwin and Jamison textbook, *Manic-Depressive Illness* (Carlson, 2007a, 2007b; Goodwin & Jamison, 2007).

In a recent article about the high reported rates of pediatric bipolar disorder in child psychiatric inpatients, Carlson was critical of interpreting irritability symptoms of childhood disorders as an expression of childhood bipolar disorder.

Impulse control deficits and affective instability in young people is now often conceptualized as bipolar disorder. However, there is broad, recognition that . . . this presentation . . . differs from BD [bipolar disorder] seen in adults. . . . Euphoria, expansiveness, supreme self-confidence, self-importance . . . are rarely seen among children. Intense, mission-driven efforts to undertake projects . . . are also rare among children. (Blader & Carlson, 2007, p. 107)

Dr. Carlson continues in this vein to note that episodes of mood disorder in children differ greatly from episodes of mood disorder in adults with bipolar disorder.

In 2006, Dr. Carlson chaired a research forum at the meeting of the American Academy of Child and Adolescent Psychiatry. The findings were published, and Dr. Carlson, who is the senior author of the article, stated,

> Impulsive, affective aggression is difficult to classify. Reframed as mood instability, it is no less complicated. Unfortunately, fitting what is likely a multitude of childhood disorders into one diagnostic category originally developed for the study of adult [bipolar disorder] remains unsatisfactory at best and destructive at worst. It is destructive both because we do not know which children are being described and thus do not know how to understand research findings, and because the valid scientific questions that have arisen have been framed in ways that cast doubt on the entire profession. (Carlson et al., 2009, p. 4)

Dr. Carlson has the well-deserved trust of a large segment of child psychiatry about bipolar disorder in children and adolescents; her beliefs about it are highly influential in the field. If she has begun to doubt the diagnosis of pediatric bipolar disorder, it likely has a poor prognosis.

REFERENCES

Biederman, J. (1995). Developmental subtypes of juvenile bipolar disorder. *Harv Rev Psychiatry, 3*(4), 227–230.

Biederman, J., Faraone, S. V., Chu, M. P., & Wozniak, J. (1999). Further evidence of a bidirectional overlap between juvenile mania and conduct disorder in children. *J Am Acad Child Adolesc Psychiatry, 38*(4), 468–476.

Biederman, J., Petty, C. R., Monuteaux, M. C., Evans, M., Parcell, T., Faraone, S. V., & Wozniak, J. (2009). The child behavior checklist-pediatric bipolar disorder profile predicts a subsequent diagnosis of bipolar disorder and associated impairments in ADHD youth growing up: A longitudinal analysis. *J Clin Psychiatry, 70*(5), 732–740.

Biederman, J., Wozniak, J., Kiely, K., Ablon, S., Faraone, S., Mick, E., Mundy E., & Kraus., I. (1995). CBCL clinical scales discriminate prepubertal children with structured interview-derived diagnosis of mania from those with ADHD. *J Am Acad Child Adolesc Psychiatry, 34*(4), 464–471.

Birmaher, B., Axelson, D., Goldstein, B., Monk, K., Kalas, C., Obreja, M., Hickey, M.B., Iyengar, S., Brent, D., Shamseddeen, W., Diler, R., & Kupfer, D. (2010). Psychiatric Disorders in Preschool Offspring of Parents With Bipolar Disorder: The Pittsburgh Bipolar Offspring Study (BIOS). *Am J Psychiatry, 167*, 321–330.

Blader, J. C., and Carlson, G. A. (2007). Increased rates of bipolar disorder diagnoses among U.S. child, adolescent, and adult inpatients, 1996–2004. *Biol Psychiatry, 62*(2), 107–114.

Carlson, G. (2007a). Children and Adolescents. In F. K. Goodwin & K. R. Jamison (Eds.) *Manic-Depressive Illness: Bipolar Disorders and Recurrent Depression.* New York: Oxford University Press.

Carlson, G. (2007b). Treatment of Children and Adolescents. In F. K. Goodwin & K. R. Jamison (Eds.) *Manic-Depressive Illness: Bipolar Disorders and Recurrent Depression.* New York: Oxford University Press.

Carlson, G. A. (2005). Early onset bipolar disorder: Clinical and research considerations. *J Clin Child Adolesc Psychol, 34*(2), 333–343.

Carlson, G. A., Findling, R. L., Post, R. M., Birmaher, B., Blumberg, H. P., Correll, C., DelBello, M. P., Fristad, M., Frazier, J., Hammen, C., Hinshaw, S. P., Kowatch, R., Leibenluft, E., Meyer, S. E., Pavuluri, M. N., Wagner, K. D., & Tohen, M. (2009). AACAP 2006 Research Forum—Advancing research in early-onset bipolar disorder: barriers and suggestions. *J Child Adolesc Psychopharmacol, 19*(1), 3–12.

Faraone, S. V., Biederman, J., Wozniak, J., Mundy, E., Mennin, D., & O'Donnell, D. (1997). Is comorbidity with ADHD a marker for juvenile-onset mania? *J Am Acad Child Adolesc Psychiatry, 36*(8), 1046–1055.

Galanter, C. A., Pagar, D. L., Oberg, P. P., Wong, C., Davies, M., & Jensen, P. S. (2009). Symptoms leading to a bipolar diagnosis: A phone survey of child and adolescent psychiatrists. *J Child Adolesc Psychopharmacol, 19*(6), 641–647.

Geller, B. (1997). Discussion of "Attention-Deficit Hyperactivity Disorder With Bipolar Disorder: A Familial Subtype?" *J. Am. Acad Child Adolesc Psychiatry, 36*(10), 1387–1388.

Geller, B., Tillman, R., & Bolhofner, K. (2007). Proposed definitions of bipolar I disorder episodes and daily rapid cycling phenomena in preschoolers, school-aged children, adolescents, and adults. *J Child Adolesc Psychopharmacol, 17*(2), 217–222.

Geller, B., Zimerman, B., Williams, M., DelBello, M., Bolhofner, K., Craney, J. L., Frazier J., Beringer L., & Nickelsburg, M. J. (2004). DSM-IV Mania Symptoms in a Prepubertal and Early Adolescent Bipolar Disorder Phenotype Compared to Attention-Deficit Hyperactive and Normal Controls. *Focus, 2,* 586–595.

Geller, B., Zimerman, B., Williams, M., Bolhofner, K, Craney, J. L., DelBello, M. P., & Soutullo, C. A. (2000). Diagnostic characteristics of 93 cases of a prepubertal and early adolescent bipolar disorder phenotype by gender, puberty and comorbid attention deficit hyperactivity disorder. *J Child Adolesc Psychopharmacol, 10*(3), 157–164.

Geller, B., Zimerman, B., Williams, M., DelBello, M. P., Frazier, J., & Beringer, L. (2002). Phenomenology of prepubertal and early adolescent bipolar disorder: examples of elated mood, grandiose behaviors, decreased need for sleep, racing thoughts and hypersexuality. *J Child Adolesc Psychopharmacol, 12*(1), 3–9.

Goodwin, F. K., & Jamison, K. R. (2007). *Manic-Depressive Illness: Bipolar Disorders and Recurrent Depression.* Oxford: Oxford University Press.

Leibenluft, E., Charney, D. S., Towbin, K. E., Bhangoo, R. K., & Pine, D. S. (2003). Defining clinical phenotypes of juvenile mania. *Am J Psychiatry, 160*(3), 430–437.

Luby, J., & Belden, A. (2006). Defining and validating bipolar disorder in the preschool period. *Dev Psychopathol, 18*(4), 971–988.

Luby, J. L., & Belden, A. C. (2008). Clinical characteristics of bipolar vs. unipolar depression in preschool children: An empirical investigation. *J Clin Psychiatry, 69*(12), 1960–1969.

McClellan, J. M., &. Speltz, M. L. (2003). Psychiatric diagnosis in preschool children. *J Am Acad Child Adolesc Psychiatry, 42*(2), 127–128; author reply, 128–130.

Safer, D. S. (2009). Irritable mood and the Diagnostic and Statistical Manual of Mental Disorders. *Child Adolesc Psychiatry Ment Health, 3.*

Singh, M. K., DelBello, M. P., Kowatch, R. A., & Strakowski, S. M. (2006). Co-occurrence of bipolar and attention-deficit hyperactivity disorders in children. *Bipolar Disord, 8*(6), 710–720.

Speltz, M. L., McClellan, J., DeKlyen, M., & Jones, K. (1999). Preschool boys with oppositional defiant disorder: Clinical presentation and diagnostic change. *J Am Acad Child Adolesc Psychiatry, 38*(7), 838–845.

Tillman, R., & Geller, B. (2003). Definitions of rapid, ultrarapid, and ultradian cycling and of episode duration in pediatric and adult bipolar disorders: A proposal to distinguish episodes from cycles. *J Child Adolesc Psychopharmacol, 13*(3), 267–271.

Wilens, T. E., Biederman, J., Brown, S., Tanguay, S., Monuteaux, M. C., Blake, C., & Spencer, T. J. (2002). Psychiatric comorbidity and functioning in clinically referred preschool children and school-age youths with ADHD. *J Am Acad Child Adolesc Psychiatry, 41*(3), 262–268.

Wilens, T., Biederman, J., Spencer T. J., & Monuteaux, M. (2003). Psychiatric Diagnosis in Preschool Children: In reply. *J. Am. Acad Child Adolesc Psychiatry, 42*, 128–129.

Wozniak, J., & Biederman, J. (1996). A pharmacological approach to the quagmire of comorbidity in juvenile mania. *J Am Acad Child Adolesc Psychiatry, 35*(6), 826–828.

Wozniak, J., Biederman J., Kiely K., Ablon J. S., Faraone S. V., Mundy E., & Mennin, D. (1995). Mania-like symptoms suggestive of childhood-onset bipolar disorder in clinically referred children. *J Am Acad Child Adolesc Psychiatry, 34*(7), 867–876.

Wozniak, J., Biederman, J., Kwon, A., Mick, E., Faraone, S., Orlovsky, K., Schnare, L., Cargol, C., & van Grondelle, A. (2005). How cardinal are cardinal symptoms in pediatric bipolar disorder? An examination of clinical correlates. *Biol Psychiatry, 58*(7), 583–538.

3

Some Studies of the Scientific Basis of Pediatric Bipolar Disorder

When a psychiatric diagnosis is proposed, it is hoped that it will describe an actual biological condition well enough to "carve nature at its seams" (Plato, as translated by Cooper in Cooper, 1997). Ideally, a diagnosis will describe a disorder in which there is an underlying biological difficulty that can eventually be found and measured. Because the biological basis of psychiatric disorders are poorly understood, a variety of cultural, economic, social, historical, and ethical factors have come to assume a significant role in the development of psychiatric diagnoses (Sadler, 2005). Adult manic-depressive illness, known as bipolar disorder in *DSM-IV*, was well described by Hippocrates in ancient Greece and has been studied and described periodically in adults for generations since then (Healy, 2008). Bipolar disorder does describe a disorder that exists in adults in the natural world; it does "carve nature at its seams." Pediatric bipolar disorder, in contrast, does not.

The criteria necessary to establish the existence of a diagnosis were described in 1970 in a classic paper by two leaders in American psychiatry, Eli Robins, MD, and Samuel Guze, MD (Robins & Guze, 1970), and came to be known as the "Robins-Guze criteria." The criteria were (1) careful clinical description; (2) laboratory studies; (3) delimitation from other disorders; (4) follow-up studies; and (5) family studies.

In the previous chapter it was argued that pediatric bipolar disorder fails to meet the first criterion, careful clinical description, and the third criterion, delimitation from other disorders. Confusion and ambiguity about the clinical appearance of pediatric bipolar disorder are pervasive. Geller and Biederman and their colleagues disagree about its appearance, and many researchers have proposed additional descriptions of pediatric bipolar disorder. The large number of proposed clinical appearances in pediatric bipolar disorder has led to calling the diagnosis a "Tower of Babel" because there are so many different descriptions and criteria that it is difficult to know what is meant (Ghaemi & Martin, 2007). The variety of clinical descriptions and the vigorous disputes they stir between researchers of the disorder strongly support the contention that the first Robins-Guze criterion for good clinical description has not been met. It is reasonable to expect that a good clinical description would lead to considerable agreement amongst those who are familiar with the disorder. This has not happened with pediatric bipolar disorder.

Delimitation from other disorders indicates the ability to separate the proposed disorder from other diagnoses. It has been discussed that it is very difficult to tell the difference between pediatric bipolar disorder and the combined diagnoses of ADHD and ODD. The demonstrated similarity in symptoms between pediatric bipolar disorder and ADHD and ODD as well the large percentage of children with the diagnosis of pediatric bipolar disorder who also have ADHD support the claim that pediatric bipolar disorder has failed to meet the Robins-Guze third criterion, delimitation from other disorders.

The second Robins-Guze criterion of psychiatric laboratory tests cannot be met for pediatric bipolar disorder because there is no such test. The absence of laboratory tests for most common psychiatric disorders weakens the science of psychiatry.

To consider the fourth and fifth Robins-Guze criteria, family studies and follow-up studies, some of the evidence supporting the genetic component of bipolar disorder and some of the studies of the age of onset of bipolar disorder will be reviewed. Despite an important genetic influence that will be described for bipolar disorder, the illness is rare to nonexistent in pre-adolescent children of parents with bipolar disorder. It is inherited but starts later in life, as will be illustrated in an examination of the follow-up studies that have been conducted on young people with at least one parent who has bipolar disorder. Studies of the frequency of bipolar disorder at different ages will be reviewed to demonstrate that bipolar disorder is not found below the age of 12.

GENETICS

To understand more fully the controversy about the diagnosis of pediatric bipolar disorder, it is important to appreciate that bipolar disorder seems largely to be an inherited disorder, passed from generation to generation genetically. Many of the studies that will be discussed below provide persuasive evidence that the offspring of adults with bipolar disorder are at a higher genetic risk for developing the disorder themselves.

How strong is heredity in the development of bipolar disorder? This has been the topic of many large studies. In 1982, Elliot Gershon, MD, and colleagues at the Biological Psychiatry Branch of NIMH conducted a study to see if bipolar disorder runs in families (Gershon et al., 1982). Family members of patients with bipolar disorder were examined for the presence of psychiatric illness. The authors found that first-degree relatives—parents, adult children, brothers, and sisters—of an adult with a clearly documented case of bipolar disorder had a 4.5% rate of bipolar disorder themselves compared to a 0% rate in the first-degree relatives of people who did not have a clearly documented case of bipolar disorder. More recent studies that have followed the children of bipolar parents as they reach late adolescence or early adulthood report similar rates of approximately 5% (Lapalme, Hodgins, & LaRoche, 1997).

A recent and exceptionally interesting study examined the familial basis of bipolar disorder among 2.7 million people aged 10–52 living in Denmark (Gottesman, Laursen, Bertelsen, & Mortensen, 2010). Because all health care in Denmark is provided by the government, each time a patient is admitted to a psychiatric hospital or to outpatient psychiatric care his or her name is recorded in a registry. Though these registries are confidential, they may be accessed for research purposes. This study compared the offspring of two adults with bipolar disorder to the offspring of one bipolar adult and one nonbipolar adult. A group of offspring of parents without a psychiatric disorder was also examined as a comparison. The study found that those with two parents with bipolar disorder were 5.7 times more likely to have bipolar disorder themselves than were those with only one parent with bipolar disorder and were 51.9 times more likely than those for whom neither parent had bipolar disorder.

Based on these studies, it is reasonable to believe that bipolar disorder is genetic. But this is not as straightforward as it might seem.

First, unlike hair color, color blindness, and some medical illnesses that are inherited through a single gene, psychiatric disorders are inherited through multiple genes, which means it is difficult to isolate them. The situation is made more complicated by the fact that there may be environmental influences at play as well. Certain social or familial situations may cause genes to express themselves or become apparent clinically. In the absence of the environmental situation, the illness might never develop even though the person has genes for the disorder. For example, there are genes related to depression that may not express themselves unless there is a significant life stress; alternatively, there may be other genes for depression that express themselves even when there is no environmental stressor. Some individuals may even inherit a genetic makeup that allows them to withstand environmental stressors without ever developing depression.

Second, families with a bipolar disorder parent may simply be more chaotic, and this may explain later problems in the offspring. For example, the bipolar parent may be intermittently psychotic, violent, hospitalized, or suicidal. Depressive episodes may contribute to the parent's psychological unavailability to the child. Substance abuse disorders co-occur in 50% of adults with bipolar disorder and may further disrupt family life. For these reasons, among others, researchers are careful to not conclude that a disorder that runs in families is necessarily a genetic disorder.

Twin studies provide a stronger way of measuring the possible role of heredity in bipolar disorder. Twin studies depend upon the genetic differences between monozygotic twins and dizygotic twins. Monozygotic twins, also called identical twins, result when a fertilized egg (zygote) splits and develops into two individuals with the same genetic makeup. They have identical genes because the embryos develop only after the fertilization of a single egg by a single sperm. With dizygotic twins, also called fraternal twins, two eggs are fertilized by two sperm at about the same time. They do not have identical genes; they share the same number of genes as do non-twin siblings.

Summarizing six studies of twin pairs in which at least one twin had bipolar disorder, Goodwin and Jamison report that 77% of the monozygotic co-twins also had the illness, compared to only 23% of the dizygotic co-twins (Goodwin & Jamison, 2007c). This strongly supports a genetic basis for bipolar disorder, although, again, there may be other explanations. Identical twins may be treated more similarly when they are growing up, particularly because they look alike and are always the same gender, which is not the case for dizygotic twins.

Given the evidence, it seems likely that bipolar disorder does have some genetic basis. It's important to note, however, that even the offspring of a bipolar parent only have roughly a 5% chance of developing the disorder—that's 1 in 20. In addition, the apparent heritability has no implications for the age of onset of the illness, as will be discussed below. Although a child of a bipolar parent may have an increased likelihood of developing bipolar disorder eventually, it is not necessarily the case that the disorder will be manifested during childhood.

AGE OF ONSET: FAMILY STUDIES

One major research strategy for the study of pediatric bipolar disorder is to look at children who have at least one bipolar parent. It is believed, based on studies such as those discussed above, that these children are at a higher genetic risk than are children whose parents do not have the disorder; if pediatric bipolar disorder does exist, these are the children in whom it ought to be found. This strategy has been used several times in the study of pediatric bipolar disorder with similar results.

In a prospective study, the questions are formulated at the beginning of the study and the children of a bipolar parent are compared over many years of development to the children without a bipolar parent. One major prospective study was undertaken by Marian Radke-Yarrow, PhD, a distinguished child development researcher from the National Institute of Mental Health. Although the study is "old"—findings were published initially in 1992—it predates the current controversies about pediatric bipolar disorder and has the great advantage of a large degree of immunity from the bias generated by the controversies (Radke-Yarrow, Nottelmann, Martinez, Fox, & Belmont, 1992). In addition, the participants in the study have been followed carefully, and reports of their functioning into young adulthood continue to be published in the current scientific literature (Meyer et al., 2004).

One hundred families participated in the original 1992 study. Each family was required to have two children, one between the ages of one and a half and three and a half and one between the ages of five and eight. Sixty-three of these families had one parent with an affective (mood) disorder, either depression or bipolar disorder. Among this group were 5 parents with bipolar disorder, 17 parents with "bipolar II" disorder (a mild form of bipolar disorder), and 41 with nonbipolar depression. The remaining 37 families were normal control families in which neither parent suffered from a psychiatric condition.

The families were assessed two different times, several years apart. In the initial assessment each of the 1½- to 3½-year-olds was examined by a psychiatrist using a wide variety of tests specific for this young age range. For example, the psychiatrist would challenge the child with brief tasks during a videotaped interview to measure the child's response to separating from the mother and the child's response to the interviewer's requests to put toys away. Based on the tests, children were rated on a number of symptoms including depression, disruptive behavior, and other behaviors. The older children, aged 5 to 8, along with their parents were given a series of diagnostic questions known as a structured psychiatric interview. Parents were also interviewed at length about their children, and they completed the Child Behavior Checklist (CBCL), a questionnaire described earlier. These procedures were repeated at the second assessment period, when the younger siblings were aged 5 to 8 years and the older siblings were aged 8 to 12 years. The considerable effort to assess the children in this study contrasts with the decision to forego interviewing the subjects in many more recent psychiatric studies of pediatric bipolar disorder.

In general, the findings indicated that the children of depressed and bipolar parents had more psychiatric problems than did the children of parents without a psychiatric condition. There was some variation by the age range of the children and also by the parents' diagnosis. For example, children of bipolar parents at age 1½ to 3½ years and 5 to 6 years had less anxiety, separated from their parents more easily, and responded less fearfully to strangers than the children of the normal or depressed parents. In the 8–11 year age range the children of bipolar parents were more often anxious than the children of the normal parents. Finally, the children of the bipolar and depressed parents had greater persistence of their problems through the age ranges studied than did the children of the normal parents. Of great interest, despite all of these careful assessments in this at-risk population, is that none of the children in any of the groups had bipolar disorder before the age of 12.

In another study by the Radke-Yarrow group, the children from the first study were assessed at regular intervals into young adulthood. In adolescence, there were no cases of mania or bipolar disorder, but there were six cases of a mild form of mania called bipolar II disorder. In young adulthood, nine offspring met criteria for bipolar I or bipolar II disorder. The diagnosis of bipolar disorder and bipolar II disorder occurred both in offspring of parents with bipolar disorder and offspring of parents with depression (Meyer et al., 2004). The results of this carefully done prospective study are consistent with the traditional understanding of pediatric bipolar disorder: there are no cases during childhood, a few in adolescence, and an increased frequency in adulthood.

Another prospective study found similar results; this study was unique in that it looked only at Amish children. This study is particularly interesting because the Amish are insulated from the world of media. Living in small rural communities, the Amish prohibit the use of most modern technologies, including electricity and automobiles. Transportation is horse drawn. The Amish culture is not influenced by the *20/20*, *Oprah*, and *Time* magazine descriptions of bipolar disorder that have inundated contemporary culture. The Amish provide an unusual opportunity to study bipolar disorder in a culture that is relatively free of media influences. Although the Amish insulate themselves from some modern aspects of the world, they are generally open to advances in contemporary medicine and have collaborated in psychiatric genetic studies of bipolar disorder and other medical conditions. The large families and lack of geographic mobility make the Amish ideal prospects for long-term study of the development of psychopathology and other illnesses in children.

The Amish study for bipolar disorder, overseen by Janice Egeland, PhD, began in 1976 with a research grant from NIMH (Egeland, Hostetter, Pauls, & Sussex, 2000; Egeland et al., 2003). Egeland and her colleagues have reported on their studies of this population over the years. This particular portion of the study was initiated in 1994, and the sample of 210 children consisted of 100 children with one parent diagnosed with bipolar disorder and 110 children with no parent diagnosed with bipolar disorder. The researchers were especially interested in studying symptoms that might predict the development of bipolar disorder, and they created an interview format specifically with this idea in mind. In order to avoid prejudging which symptoms might predict future bipolar disorder, they collected information about a wide array of symptoms.

The findings of the study are particularly interesting for two reasons: First, none of the children 12 and below had bipolar disorder. Second, the symptoms that characterized the young children's difficulties were not those that most often describe pediatric bipolar disorder in the recent research literature. The children of Amish parents with bipolar disorder did not have the intense disruptive behaviors of the bipolar children described by Beiderman and Geller (Egeland et al., 2003). Amongst the many symptoms found in the prepubertal children of an Amish parent with bipolar disorder were "withdrawal, apathy, underactivity, anxious/worried, and attention problems/distractible." Although there was some evidence that the problems of these children fluctuated in severity, the symptoms were not similar to the irritability described by the Biederman group nor the grandiosity and elation described by the Geller group. In fact, the children of the Amish normal control parents had a greater tendency to exhibit "grand/lots of ideas, conduct problems, and bed wetting" than did the children of the parents with bipolar disorder.

As the children grew into adolescence, they tended to become hyperactive and irritable, and with age, some developed bipolar disorder. When the children of bipolar parents were aged 13–27, two had developed bipolar disorder and two had developed bipolar II disorder (Egeland, Shaw, Endicott, Allen, & Hostetter, 2005). Once again, this prospective study confirms a classical view of bipolar disorder: pediatric bipolar disorder in children before puberty is absent. Cases begin to appear in adolescence and early adulthood at a rate of roughly 4–5%.

Anne Duffy, MD, a psychiatric researcher at the University of Ottawa, has recently reviewed several studies that prospectively follow high-risk children of parents with bipolar disorder and reports that none of the offspring who eventually developed bipolar disorder developed it as children (Duffy, 2007). Not finding pediatric bipolar disorder before the age of 13 in these children of a bipolar parent studied as they grew up is strong evidence that the disorder does not exist in children. Duffy's review is also noteworthy for not finding significant amounts of ADHD in the offspring of the bipolar parents. Duffy's own longitudinal study of children born to one parent with bipolar disorder over a 15-year period failed to uncover a single case of bipolar disorder during the childhood of the bipolar offspring she followed (Duffy, 2009).

Based on her own longitudinal study and those she reviewed, Duffy has proposed several stages in the development of bipolar disorder. Looking back on children who eventually develop the disorder as adults, these are the childhood symptoms that most often preceded adult bipolar disorder. As young children, they tended to have sleep difficulties and anxiety, which was then followed in some by mild depression. During adolescence, some developed depression and finally, as adults, bipolar disorder (Duffy, 2009).

Once again, the children depicted in the pre-illness phases of the development of bipolar disorder described by Duffy have nothing in common with the bipolar children of Biederman or Geller and their colleagues. They are not irritable, grandiose, or enraged. Nor do they have ADHD. Whatever may be wrong with the children discussed by the Biederman and Geller groups, it is not consistent with the appearance of bipolar disorder found in the longitudinal studies of offspring of bipolar parents. It is a different disorder entirely (Goodwin & Jamison, 2007b).

AGE OF ONSET: SELF-REPORT

In addition to the prospective studies outlined above, there are also several frequently discussed retrospective studies. Retrospective studies attempt to determine when bipolar disorder begins by asking adult patients to recall when their symptoms began. These studies, which have been very influential and are frequently cited in the professional literature, have reported that the disorder often begins in children under the age of 12. Although the studies are flawed in that they are based on recall rather than observation, they have nonetheless served to provide a rationale for making the diagnosis of pediatric bipolar disorder.

In one such study, Lish and colleagues (Lish, Dime-Meenan, Whybrow, Price, & Hirschfeld, 1994) surveyed adult members of the National Depressive and Manic-Depressive Association (DMDA) who currently had bipolar disorder and asked the age at which the symptoms were first experienced. The DMDA is a national patient-run organization that advocates for research and clinical care for depression and bipolar disorder. Of the 500 survey responses that were received, 5% of the patients reported that the symptoms began younger than the age of 5 years; 12% reported that the symptoms began between the ages of 5 years and 9 years; 14% reported that the symptoms began between the ages of 10 years and 14 years; 28% reported that the symptoms began between the ages of 15 years and 19 years; and 40% reported that the symptoms began at age 20 or later.

There are many problems with this study, and it would be an error to conclude that bipolar disorder begins before the age of 14 for almost one-third of patients. First, the patients were not asked to date the onset of their full illness but only to report the onset of individual symptoms listed in the survey. Many of these symptoms, such as depressed mood, anger, and lack of sleep, could be attributed to a variety of other psychiatric disorders.

Second, like all retrospective studies, the data are based on memory and patient self-report and are therefore subject to a considerable amount of unwitting distortion by the patient. The development of a major medical or psychiatric illness can lead a patient to recall the past in a way that makes it more in accordance with the current situation. For example, a patient with newly diagnosed diabetes might begin to selectively remember all the times he or she ate excessive forbidden sweets during childhood. These memories might achieve a prominence they had not had before the diabetes diagnosis, and in fact the memories of eating sweets might become exaggerated. Similarly, if a patient develops bipolar disorder, the patient might re-interpret his or her childhood to align memories of it with the knowledge of the newly diagnosed illness. Such patients may interpret normal behaviors of childhood as "bipolar symptoms" once the diagnosis is part of the patient's current experience. The past of course cannot be altered, but the understanding, interpretation, and recollection of it by patients changes with time and present events. In this sense, at least, the present changes the past. Patient self-reports of the past should not be taken by physicians and researchers as factual. The rates of bipolar disorder in children below the age of 14 in these studies far exceed by many times the rates reported in more carefully done studies (Burke, Burke, Regier, & Rae, 1990).

In terms of the Robins-Guze criteria, the follow-up studies and family studies do not support the existence of bipolar disorder in children under the age of 12.

EPIDEMIOLOGY

Stated most simply, epidemiology is concerned with the study of illness among populations. Epidemiologists may look for the number of cases of a given illness in a certain geographic area, among a certain group of people exposed to a certain drug, among a certain age group, or among people who were exposed to a certain catastrophic event such as an earthquake or the 9/11 disaster. Epidemiologists were the first to notice the association between cigarette smoking and lung cancer. It was a group of epidemiologists who first reported the sudden and dramatic forty-fold increase in the diagnosis of outpatient pediatric bipolar disorder (Moreno et al., 2007).

The importance of epidemiology is often illustrated by describing one of the cases of a pioneer in the field. In the mid-1800s, London was beset by a catastrophic epidemic of cholera, a fatal and highly contagious disease. No one knew what caused the disease or how it was spread. John Snow, the father of epidemiology, believed that it might be caused by contaminated drinking water. By carefully plotting the homes of all of the known cholera patients onto a map of London and also plotting which areas of the city were served by which water companies, he was able to show that a certain water company was providing the water to all of the areas in which the infected people lived. By improving the hand-washing behaviors of the employees of the water company, he ended the epidemic.

Psychiatric epidemiology, unlike the epidemiology of other diseases, cannot rely on blood tests or other biological means of counting illness cases. Instead, psychiatric epidemiologists typically interview patients or those who care for patients. The need for psychiatric epidemiologists to have recognized criteria to diagnose various psychiatric illnesses, in fact, was an important motivation for the development of the *DSM* system.

Counting the number of psychiatrically ill people in the United States has been a challenge. Such estimates are important because they help shape health care budgets, insurance company rates, and resources allocated to treat and care for mentally ill people.

How many adults have bipolar disorder? Summarizing six of the most ambitious and carefully done epidemiologic studies of psychiatric disorders in adults, Goodwin and Jamison report that these studies considered together suggest that 1% of the U.S. adult population has bipolar disorder (Costello et al., 1996; Goodwin & Jamison, 2007b). The recent large increase in the number of cases of pediatric bipolar disorder diagnosed in treatment settings is inconsistent with the 1% prevalence found in adulthood.

Once bipolar disorder emerges, it lasts throughout life. If 1% of the adult population have bipolar disorder, the childhood rate of 5% advanced by the proponents of pediatric bipolar disorder cannot be correct. It is clearly an overestimate; the reported rate in children far exceeds the rate in adults, which is not plausible.

The epidemiology of pediatric bipolar disorder is murky due to a relative absence of national studies on the subject. The single major epidemiological study of psychiatric disorders in childhood in the United States was conducted by Dr. Jane Costello and colleagues and used a limited geographic area, the Smoky Mountains of North Carolina (Costello et al., 1996). The participants included 1,420 children aged 9–16 years who were selected to represent the children of North Carolina. The children entered the study between the ages of 9 and 13 years and were assessed annually until age 16. Over the three years, 36.7% of the children had received some form of psychiatric diagnosis (this includes a wide array of relatively benign disorders such as bedwetting and fears). The findings also showed that during any three-month period, 13.3% of the children had one of these diagnoses. Amongst the many interesting findings in this carefully done study was that the frequency of psychiatric illness in children declined from age 9 to 12 but began to climb again with the onset of adolescence. Despite the exhaustive documentation of the problems of childhood, not a single case of bipolar disorder was identified.

Noting the absence of epidemiological studies in the United States, an international group of psychiatrists surveyed the rates of bipolar disorder in children outside of the United States (Soutullo et al., 2005). The group reported a major epidemiological study in England that did not find any cases of pediatric bipolar disorder. Remarkably, of 2,500 referrals of children under the age of 10 to a university medical center in England, there was not a single case of bipolar disorder. Soutullo and colleagues also discussed an epidemiologic study done in Holland of adolescents aged 13 to 18 years that found a 1.9% prevalence of mania (Verhulst, van der Ende, Ferdinand, & Kasius, 1997). Reviewing the percentage of children and adolescents diagnosed with bipolar disorder in clinics and inpatient units across Europe, Soutullo and colleagues noted that, in general, the rates were low as compared to those in the United States. They conclude that the discrepancy between rates in the United States and those in Europe may be due to a variety of factors, including the differences in criteria used to determine the disorder.

This seemed to be the case in a separate study that was conducted by psychiatrists from England and the United States who were working in collaboration. There is an admirable precedent of international scientific collaboration between psychiatrists in England and the United States. In situations in which the two groups diagnose similar patients differently, they have performed studies together to assess the reasons for the differences so as to consider amending diagnostic practices as seems appropriate. As noted, the English rarely if ever diagnose bipolar disorder in children below the age of 12, yet the practice is common in the United States. To study this further, five brief written case histories of children who might have bipolar disorder were developed collaboratively by psychiatrists from both countries. One case described a 12-year-old girl who clearly had all of the symptoms of bipolar disorder, and both the U.S. and English psychiatrists agreed on the diagnosis. In the other four cases the diagnosis was much more ambiguous. Perhaps not surprisingly, the psychiatrists in the United States diagnosed bipolar disorder often in these ambiguous cases; the English psychiatrists did not. The English psychiatrists did not even consider the possibility that the children might have bipolar disorder. This is especially interesting given the fact that the psychiatrists from both countries recognized and agreed upon the symptoms that were described for all of the children. The difference in diagnosis hinged on their interpretation of those symptoms. The study lends support for the well-recognized propensity for U.S. psychiatrists to diagnose pediatric bipolar disorder when psychiatrists in other countries would not (Dubicka, Carlson, Vail, & Harrington, 2008).

TREATMENT OR PREVENTION?

One possible explanation for the U.S. propensity to diagnose bipolar disorder in children is the notion that doing so could serve to prevent what would otherwise be a more serious case of the disorder later.

This belief stems from the "kindling theory" of Robert Post, MD, a distinguished scholar at NIMH. Dr. Post proposed that each manic episode of bipolar disorder predisposes the brain to have a subsequent episode more quickly. The theory is based on findings about rats that were administered electric stimulation to the brain: When rats are given sufficient electrical stimulation they will have seizures. Over time, less and less electrical stimulation will cause a seizure—the brain has become "sensitized" (reacts more quickly) to the stimulation. This is compared to adding kindling so that a fire starts more quickly—hence the name "kindling theory" (Goddard, 1967). According to the kindling theory, preventing a manic episode is like preventing an episode of electric stimulation to a rat brain; the theory is that each manic episode makes it easier for the patient to have another manic episode. If you prevent a manic episode in a child, according to the theory, you might prevent future episodes from occurring (Post, 2009). It was even speculated that preventing an episode might prevent actual brain damage.

The theory had some support by the observation that the time between episodes of bipolar disorder in adult patients shortened for at least the first few episodes in many studies. Recent evidence, however, has not lent support to the kindling theory, as the time between episodes does not always shorten with each episode (Goodwin & Jamison, 2007a). The kindling theory in adult bipolar disorder is an interesting idea with mixed scientific support that nonetheless has been very influential in pediatric bipolar disorder.

The prevention of mental illness is a major goal for child psychiatry and other child mental health disciplines. This goal remains elusive. Although prevention is written about with regard to pediatric bipolar disorder, the issue is especially difficult to address clinically because of controversies about diagnosing and treating the disorder that are unresolved. An important subtext of the interest in pediatric bipolar disorder over the past 20 years is the implicit hope that by identifying and treating prepubertal forms of the disorder the onset of the destructive adult form with its suicidality and psychiatric hospitalizations might be prevented. As argued, this seems to have had the unintended consequence of diagnosing many children with the disorder when they didn't have it and of depriving those children of effective treatments for the disorders they did have.

One of the many ambiguities in the preventive aspect of the pediatric bipolar disorder initiative is distinguishing between preventing the illness before signs and symptoms of it appear and treating the illness after it has appeared. Is treating pediatric bipolar disorder a treatment effort or a prevention effort?

Preventing an illness before signs and symptoms appear is known as primary prevention. For pediatric bipolar disorder, this form of prevention carries risks: a large number of children may be labeled and treated despite the fact that most would never have developed the disorder. Even if the intervention is targeted to those most at risk—the children of a bipolar parent, for example—95% of the children would never have developed the disorder even as adults.

Children of bipolar parents who develop symptoms of behavior disorders and/or depression are often treated differently from other children with the same symptoms in the belief that doing so represents prevention of later adult bipolar disorder (Chang, 2008). Focusing treatment on the prevention of future bipolar disorder, however, may unnecessarily lead to withholding medications that might be very helpful to these children, including stimulants for the treatment of ADHD and antidepressants for the treatment of depression. The concern about a diagnosis the child might have in the future can obscure recognition of current diagnoses and inhibit the clearly indicated treatments of the diagnoses from which the child suffers in the immediate present. This is not to suggest that the risks of the potential development of bipolar disorder should be ignored; rather, these risks and their reduction should be considered along with all the other risks and benefits of the medications for treating the patient's current illness.

REFERENCES

Burke, K.C., Burke, J.D. Jr., Regier, D.A., & Rae, D.S. (1990). Age at onset of selected mental disorders in five community populations. *Arch Gen Psychiatry, 47*(6), 511–518.

Chang, K. (2008). Treatment of Children and Adolescents at High Risk for Bipolar Disorder. In B. Geller & M.P. DelBello (Eds.), *Treatment of Bipolar Disorder in Children and Adolescents* (pp. 287–305). New York: The Guilford Press.

Cooper, J.M. (1997). *The Complete Works of Plato.* Indianapolis: Hacket.

Costello, E.J., Angold, A., Burns, B.J., Stangl, D.K., Tweed, D.L., Erkanli, A., et al. (1996). The Great Smoky Mountains Study of Youth. Goals, design, methods, and the prevalence of DSM-III-R disorders. *Arch Gen Psychiatry, 53*(12), 1129–1136.

Dubicka, B., Carlson, G.A., Vail, A., & Harrington, R. (2008). Prepubertal mania: diagnostic differences between U.S. and UK clinicians. *Eur Child Adolesc Psychiatry, 17*(3), 153–161.

Duffy, A. (2007). Does bipolar disorder exist in children? A selected review. *Can J Psychiatry, 52*(7), 409–417.

Duffy, A. (2009). The early course of bipolar disorder in youth at familial risk. *J Can Acad Child Adolesc Psychiatry, 18*(3), 200–205.

Egeland, J.A., Hostetter, A.M., Pauls, D.L., & Sussex, J.N. (2000). Prodromal symptoms before onset of manic-depressive disorder suggested by first hospital admission histories. *J Am Acad Child Adolesc Psychiatry, 39*(10), 1245–1252.

Egeland, J.A., Shaw, J.A., Endicott, J., Pauls, D.L., Allen, C.R., Hostetter, A.M., et al. (2003). Prospective study of prodromal features for bipolarity in well Amish children. *J Am Acad Child Adolesc Psychiatry, 42*(7), 786–796.

Egeland, J.A., Shaw, J.A., MD, Endicott, P.D., Allen, C., BA, & Hostetter, A. M. (2005). In Response. *Journal of the American Academy of Child and Adolescent Psychiatry, 44*(11), 1115–1117.

Gershon, E.S., Hamovit, J., Guroff, J.J., Dibble, E., Leckman, J.F., Sceery, W., et al. (1982). A family study of schizoaffective, bipolar I, bipolar II, unipolar, and normal control probands. *Arch Gen Psychiatry, 39*(10), 1157–1167.

Ghaemi, S. N., & Martin, A. (2007). Defining the boundaries of childhood bipolar disorder. *Am J Psychiatry, 164*(2), 185–188.

Goddard, G. V. (1967). Development of epileptic seizures through brain stimulation at low intensity. *Nature, 214*(5092), 1020–1021.

Goodwin, F. K., & Jamison, K. R. (2007a). Clinical Studies-Course and Outcome. In F. K. Goodwin & K. R. Jamison (Eds.), *Manic-Depressive Illness: Bipolar Disorders and Recurrent Depression.* Oxford: Oxford University Press.

Goodwin, F. K., & Jamison, K. R. (2007b). Epidemiology-Community Surveys among Adults. In F. K. Goodwin & J. K. Redfield (Eds.), *Manic-Depressive Illness: Bipolar Disorders and Recurrent Depression.* Oxford: Oxford University Press.

Goodwin, F. K., & Jamison, K. R. (2007c). Twin Studies. In F. Goodwin & K. R. Jamison (Eds.), *Manic-Depressive Illness* (pp. 419–420). Oxford: Oxford University Press.

Gottesman, I. I., Laursen, T. M., Bertelsen, A., & Mortensen, P. B. (2010). Severe mental disorders in offspring with 2 psychiatrically ill parents. *Arch Gen Psychiatry, 67*(3), 252–257.

Healy, D. (2008). Frenzy and Stupor. In D. Healy (Ed.), *Mania: A Short History of Bipolar Disorder* (pp. 1–23). Baltimore: The Johns Hopkins University Press.

Lapalme, M., Hodgins, S., & LaRoche, C. (1997). Children of parents with bipolar disorder: A metaanalysis of risk for mental disorders. *Can J Psychiatry, 42*(6), 623–631.

Lish, J. D., Dime-Meenan, S., Whybrow, P. C., Price, R. A., & Hirschfeld, R. M. (1994). The National Depressive and Manic-depressive Association (DMDA) survey of bipolar members. *J Affect Disord, 31*(4), 281–294.

Meyer, S. E., Carlson, G. A., Wiggs, E. A., Martinez, P. E., Ronsaville, D. S., Klimes-Dougan, B., et al. (2004). A prospective study of the association among impaired executive functioning, childhood attentional problems, and the development of bipolar disorder. *Dev Psychopathol, 16*(2), 461–476.

Moreno, C., Laje, G., Blanco, C., Jiang, H., Schmidt, A. B., & Olfson, M. (2007). National trends in the outpatient diagnosis and treatment of bipolar disorder in youth. *Arch Gen Psychiatry, 64*(9), 1032–1039.

Post, R. M. (2009). Sensitization Phenomena Emphasizing the Need for Early Treatment. In R. A. Kowatch, M. A. Fristad, R. L. Findling, & P.R.M. (Eds.), *Clinical Manual for Management of Bipolar Disorder in Children and Adolescents.* Arlington: American Psychiatric Publishing, Inc.

Radke-Yarrow, M., Nottelmann, E., Martinez, P., Fox, M. B., & Belmont, B. (1992). Young children of affectively ill parents: a longitudinal study of psychosocial development. *J Am Acad Child Adolesc Psychiatry, 31*(1), 68–77.

Robins, E., & Guze, S. B. (1970). Establishment of diagnostic validity in psychiatric illness: its application to schizophrenia. *Am J Psychiatry, 126*(7), 983–987.

Sadler, J. Z. (2005). *Values and Psychiatric Diagnosis.* Oxford: Oxford University Press.

Soutullo, C. A., Chang, K. D., Diez-Suarez, A., Figueroa-Quintana, A., Escamilla-Canales, I., Rapado-Castro, M., et al. (2005). Bipolar disorder in children and adolescents: International perspective on epidemiology and phenomenology. *Bipolar Disord, 7*(6), 497–506.

Verhulst, F. C., van der Ende, J., Ferdinand, R. F., & Kasius, M. C. (1997). The prevalence of DSM-III-R diagnoses in a national sample of Dutch adolescents. *Arch Gen Psychiatry, 54*(4), 329–336.

4

Cultural Influences in Pediatric Bipolar Disorder

During my psychiatry residency, I was fortunate to attend a series of lectures on research methods by Martin Orne, MD, a distinguished research psychiatrist. Dr. Orne was interested in studying the nature of hypnosis. He was especially interested in the question of whether a hypnotic trance was an actual biological state or was simply role-play or acting. In the late 1800s, when hypnosis was a popular entertainment, theaters regularly booked stage hypnotists to perform before large audiences. Inevitably, part of the performance included putting the entire audience in a trance. The hypnotist would ask the audience members to close their eyes and relax. More often than not, as the audience entered the trance state, they would slowly raise their right hands without being asked or told to do so. There is nothing about entering a trance state that has anything to do with raising your right hand, yet the audience—based on what they had heard, read, or seen about hypnosis—believed that you were supposed to raise your right hand. They did not have to be told to do this. It was part of the culture; they knew it, and they complied with cultural expectations.

It is my contention that something similar has happened with pediatric bipolar disorder. Culture influences every aspect of this disorder—from its adoption as a valid diagnosis to the dramatic rise in the number of cases in the decade following its introduction. This chapter will discuss the role culture plays in the creation and expression of mental illness and explore some of the events in the culture that contributed to the sudden rise of the pediatric bipolar disorder diagnosis.

HOW CULTURE HELPS SHAPE MENTAL ILLNESS

Most American psychiatrists believe that mental illness exists as a physiological state that is largely beyond the realm of social or cultural influence. The *DSM-IV* defines mental illness as occurring *inside* the person (American Psychiatric Association, 2000). Mental illness as a physical disease is a critical presupposition in the *DSM*, and this leaves little room for the role of culture in the study of psychiatric illness. As journalist Ethan Watters notes in a *New York Times* article titled "The Americanization of Mental Illness," the *DSM-IV* relegates the influence of culture to an appendix of *DSM-IV* in which a variety of odd behavioral syndromes found in non-Western societies creates a "carnival sideshow" for the curious visitor (Watters, 2010a). Although some attention is paid to culture in non-Western countries, the *DSM-IV* simply does not address the pervasive and powerful influence of culture in the diagnosis and treatment of mental illness in the United States.

Despite being de-emphasized in the *DSM-IV*, culture has always had an influence on psychopathology. Diagnostic rates rise and fall de-pending on the culture's view of a particular illness at a particular point in time. The fact that there seem to be trends in psychopathology is in no way meant to diminish the suffering of those who are mentally ill. It simply means that the way an individual's suffering is expressed is open to influence by popular culture. For example, at the end of the 19th century and into the early part of the 20th century "conversion reactions"—also known as "hysteria"—were among the more widely discussed psychiatric disorders. Patients suffering from conversion reactions would display neurological symptoms, such as loss of sight or paralysis, with no apparent underlying physical cause. Though "conversion disorder" still remains in the *DSM-IV*, it is generally considered to have disappeared by the end of the 20th century and is rarely diagnosed today. Several decades ago, when multiple personality disorder became a subject of media attention and was portrayed in several books and films, there was a marked increase in the number of psychiatric patients who displayed those symptoms.

Similarly, in the early 1990s, when the sexual abuse of children was a focus of media attention, a proliferation of cases of "repressed memories" of sexual abuse in early infancy were recalled suddenly by adults under hypnosis, and the subject of repressed memory appeared frequently in the psychiatric and lay literature (Loftus & J. E., 1995). Cases of conversion reactions, multiple personality disorder, and repressed memory syndrome have decreased considerably in the recent past, which supports the idea that they were tied to the amount of media attention they received.

Much of American culture exerts its influence through media— television, movies, the Internet, newspapers, magazines, and books— and many form knowledge and beliefs about mental illness from the information received from these sources. The direct marketing of psychiatric diagnoses in the guise of educating the public about the illnesses is a practice that pharmaceutical companies have been alleged to use to increase the rates of psychiatric illness recognized by the consumers. The pharmaceutical companies believe that customers will use the company's medication to treat the advertised illnesses. This practice, called "disease mongering" exemplifies the media creation of an illness (Moynihan & Henry, 2006).

In the *New York Times* article mentioned above, Watters discusses the effect media can have on how mental illness is experienced and identified within a culture. Citing the work of the medical historian Edward Shorter, Watters explains that each culture identifies its own "symptom repertoire," described as a unique array of symptoms that express mental illness in that particular culture. Individuals who are suffering express their pain using symptoms from the repertoire of their culture. This is not done consciously. When a new diagnosis is created by professionals and disseminated by the media, it enters the symptom repertoire and becomes available for selection by suffering members of the culture. In this way, according to Watters, simply proposing a new psychiatric diagnosis can lead to an increase in the number of patients who then get those symptoms.

As an example of this phenomenon, Watters cites the dramatic rise in the number of cases of anorexia nervosa in Hong Kong following the introduction of the diagnosis by the media (Watters, 2010b). Anorexia nervosa is a well-known psychiatric disorder in the United States. Most frequently, the disorder begins in young female adolescents who have a distorted view of themselves as fat and use very restrictive diets and intense exercise to lose weight. In extreme cases, starved and emaciated, they continue to lose weight and may die. Prior to 1994, there were virtually no cases of this type of anorexia nervosa in Hong Kong. Instead, there were rare cases of a form of anorexia in which girls had a sense of fullness, pain, and pressure in their stomachs and throats and decreased their eating, but they did not think they were fat, did not want to lose weight, and did not intentionally diet or exercise. Then, in November 1994, a young Chinese woman died suddenly of anorexia. The Hong Kong media began reporting on the illness for the first time, often copying symptoms of "American-style" anorexia nervosa directly from the *DSM-IV*. Following this media attention there was a sudden and dramatic increase in the number of American-style anorexia patients in Hong Kong. This cultural phenomenon led to the serious illness of many young women.

Many psychiatrists believe that a rise in the number of cases of a newly introduced disorder is due to an increased recognition of a disorder by psychiatrists and other health care professionals that existed previously but was not identified. In contrast, Watters believes that the announcement of the disorder can actually *create* the diagnosis, as it did in Hong Kong. When a society's "symptom repertoire" increases to include a new illness, those symptoms become available as a choice for individuals who are suffering.

A similar dynamic may have contributed to the dramatic rise in the rates of diagnosed pediatric bipolar disorder in the United States. Many children are unruly and difficult to manage. If one considers the arguments outlined above, it is easy to see how the explosion in media coverage of the pediatric bipolar disorder diagnosis may have led to the actual creation of new cases of the disorder. Watters's case for this in Hong Kong is persuasive. My own experience and that of other psychiatrists with a flood of parents complaining that their children had "mood swings" and were convinced their children had bipolar disorder, along with the media attention the disorder received, supports this possibility.

Watters's observations and theories underscore the risk that publicizing a disorder can lead to an increase in the number of new cases. This seems much closer to the truth of the matter than simply attributing the dramatic rise in cases to an increased recognition of the disorder. At the very least it suggests that some caution might be exercised before announcing the birth of a new disorder. Such a warning might be particularly timely on the eve of the release of the new *DSM-V* (Yan, 2010) when it can be expected that the "symptom repertoire" will increase as the public learns of many new psychiatric diagnoses.

PEDIATRIC BIPOLAR DISORDER AS A MEDIA EVENT

The media debut of pediatric bipolar disorder began with the publication of the book *The Bipolar Child* by Demitri Papolos, MD, and Janice Papolos, a husband-and-wife team (Papolos & Papolos, 2006). Dr. Papolos, an adult psychiatrist, is an associate professor of psychiatry at the Albert Einstein College of Medicine and codirects its program in behavioral genetics. He has received funding from both the National Institute of Mental Health and the National Alliance for Research on Schizophrenia and Depression. He is not a child psychiatrist. Janice

Papolos is a medical writer who has coauthored several books including another best-selling mental health self-help book, *Overcoming Depression*, which she also wrote with her husband. *The Bipolar Child* is among the most influential popular press books written in the field of child mental health, perhaps because it purports to offer help for a very difficult group of children. The media attention it received certainly boosted its popularity as well. As part of its initial promotion, the Papoloses were featured on the national network television program *20/20*. Within 30 minutes of the segment's airing, *20/20* received more than 6,000 e-mails. Soon after, the authors were featured on several other highly visible television shows, including *The Oprah Winfrey Show*, the CBS *Early Show*, and the CBS evening news with Dan Rather (as reported on the authors' Web site, www.bipolarchild.com).

The book was extremely well received by the reading public and has sold over 200,000 copies to date. The extensive media coverage also served as a public relations blitz for the diagnosis of pediatric bipolar disorder. The Papoloses have started two foundations, issue a newsletter with 20,000 subscribers, and operate a Web site (www.bipolarchild. com). All of these highly successful activities have also helped to create public support for the diagnosis.

At first glance *The Bipolar Child* seems to be a responsible effort to communicate the characteristics of bipolar disorder to a group of parents whose children suffer from a variety of symptoms. On closer examination, however, it becomes apparent that the effort is less helpful than it seems. The description of pediatric bipolar disorder put forth in the book bears little resemblance to the actual disorder as it is understood in the *DSM-IV*. The reader is told that a wide spectrum of symptoms found in children are due to bipolar disorder. The current edition of the book includes a parent questionnaire that lists 65 such symptoms, most of which are not associated with *DSM-IV* bipolar disorder. Among these are night terrors, separation anxiety, hoarding behavior, complaints of boredom, apathetic withdrawal, and being "very intuitive and/or creative." Another purported symptom of childhood bipolar disorder that typifies the book's indifference to established diagnostic criteria is difficulty waking up in the morning. Many children have trouble waking up in the morning, and this has no bearing on whether the children have bipolar disorder. At a conference several years ago I was surprised to hear a distinguished authority in child psychiatry confidently confirm the view that difficulty waking in the morning is symptomatic of bipolar disorder in childhood. If this everyday complaint is taken as a symptom of childhood bipolar disorder, it is easy to understand why the frequency of this diagnosis may have increased greatly over the past several years.

The book emphasizes the irritability, rages, and aggression of the bipolar child and notes that many of the children regarded as having bipolar disorder have ADHD as well. It confronts the possibility that ADHD may be difficult to distinguish from bipolar disorder in childhood but nonetheless claims to be able to do so. To make the distinction, the book reproduces a list of 12 ways to distinguish between the two diagnoses. The list was written originally by Charles Popper, MD, from Harvard University, a former editor of the *Journal of Child and Adolescent Psychopharmacology*. The statements in this list have little or no evidence to support them. They seem to be clinical speculations or guesses about what may be true, but any weight they add to the scientific basis for making the distinction between pediatric bipolar disorder and ADHD is totally unwarranted. For example, one statement (#4) reports that children who have ADHD only have temper tantrums when they are overstimulated, whereas children who have bipolar disorder have temper tantrums when they are told "no." This is not true. Oppositional defiant disorder, which frequently accompanies ADHD, is in fact characterized by difficulties taking no for an answer. It is all too common for ADHD children to have problems with this, and it hardly merits adding the diagnosis of bipolar disorder.

Similarly, the list includes a statement (#10) that misbehavior on the part of ADHD children is accidental while misbehavior in those with bipolar disorder is intentional. Again, this is not true. Children with ADHD who misbehave intentionally, and there are plenty, are best diagnosed with ODD as well as ADHD. Once more, the addition of bipolar disorder is unwarranted.

Finally, the list indicates that lithium treatment leads to improvement in bipolar disorder but not in ADHD. There is no evidence to support the contention that lithium works for bipolar disorder in children. Although there is no evidence or science supporting any of Dr. Popper's 12 recommendations for making the distinction between bipolar disorder and ADHD, the Papoloses heartily endorse the list and have nothing to add in making the distinction.

The book is resolutely optimistic, with no doubts or misgivings about its conclusions and recommendations. It makes a great effort to persuade the public that pediatric bipolar disorder is a relatively common but largely unrecognized disorder that should be identified and treated. The book also cautions the reader that the child should be treated with "mood stabilizers" early on, "before episodes become more frequent and the illness warps the psychological development of a child and destroys the life of a family" (Papolos & Papolos, 2006, p. xvi).

The perception that the disorder is widespread is encouraged by the authors' use of a Web-based methodology to gather data. Parents who believe their child has bipolar disorder—whether or not the child has received the diagnosis or even been psychiatrically evaluated—write to the Web site with descriptions of their child's behavior and get advice from other consumers and physician consultants. This is not a science-based method for learning about childhood bipolar disorder. Rather, it seems to be a good method for reinforcing the beliefs, perceptions, and fears of those who write to the Web site. It creates a cult-like atmosphere. This is reinforced when the authors advise parents who believe their child may have bipolar disorder to seek a child psychiatrist who is not strongly committed to *DSM-IV.*

Since the publication of *The Bipolar Child,* a large number of additional self-help books for parents who believe they have bipolar children have appeared, including, for example, in no particular order, *Parenting a Bipolar Child: What to Do & Why* (Faedda & Austin, 2006); *The Ups and Downs of Raising a Bipolar Child: A Survival Guide for Parents* (Lederman & Fink, 2003); and *Understanding the Mind of Your Bipolar Child: The Complete Guide to the Development, Treatment, and Parenting of Children with Bipolar Disorder* (Lombardo, 2006). All of the books strongly endorse the existence of the disorder and provide guidance for its management to distressed parents.

A disturbing variation on the self-help book for parents are books written for parents to read to their young children diagnosed with bipolar disorder. Through the skillful use of language and illustrations, the books are moving to read and do a good job of portraying the world of the troubled child. The characters' situations are more heartbreaking when it becomes apparent that the books are incorrectly concluding that the children portrayed have bipolar disorder when they do not. Healy has also described these books and their inaccuracy in diagnosing bipolar disorder (Healy, 2008).

Consider *Brandon and the Bipolar Bear: A Story for Children with Bipolar Disorder* (Anglada, Taylor, & Ferguson, 2004). The book tells the story of one day in the life of Brandon, a young boy who is put to bed but then asks for a glass of water. He feels somewhat frightened and becomes tearful when left alone to fall asleep. Upon awakening, he has a temper tantrum because he doesn't want to get out of bed. During the tantrum he tears off the arm of his beloved teddy bear. He is crushed by his destruction of his teddy bear but is greatly relieved when his mother offers to fix its arm. He becomes excited and bounces up and down on his bed. He goes to see Dr. Samuel, who tells him he has bipolar disorder and that he inherited it like the color of his hair. Dr. Samuel gives him medicine. None of Brandon's behaviors alone or together are symptoms of bipolar disorder. Dr. Samuel, the genial final authority on diagnosis and treatment in the book, seems to have let his young patient down.

Further, consider Robert in *My Bipolar Roller Coaster Feelings Book* (Hebert, Hannah, & Hebert, 2005). Robert seems remarkably free from bipolar disorder as well. ADHD and fear of the dark seem closer to his actual diagnoses. He shouts out answers in class and has to remember to raise his hand. He is very excited about school and can get overexcited and giddy when he is very happy. He has a tantrum when his mother does not get him something he wanted in a store. He is afraid of the dark and is easily frustrated. He has trouble getting organized and has brief periods of unhappiness or "depression." He works hard to control himself in school and in karate class. His doctor believes he has bipolar disorder. Robert's parents tell him at the end of the book that bipolar disorder is just a part of who he is and not all of who he is. Yet it doesn't seem to me that any part of Robert has bipolar disorder, and this diagnosis is a burden from which he could easily be relieved.

These two children's books represent everything that is so chilling about the diagnosis of pediatric bipolar disorder: the children don't have the disease; they have difficulties in their current lives that are not addressed (at least ADHD for Robert); and their views of themselves and others' views of them will be in part based on the misunderstanding of their current diagnosis. Later in life, their trust in the helping professions will be shaken when it is realized that they do not have the disorder for which they have been diagnosed and treated.

In a twist on this child-oriented genre, there are some first-person accounts in which children contribute directly to the literature on pediatric bipolar disorder. In *Bipolar Bubbles: A Positive Journey Through the Eyes of a Child with Bipolar Disorder,* the bipolar child coauthors the book with her mother (Theisen & Theisen, 2008). The story is told well and the illustrations are particularly engaging. I can't bring myself to criticize a child author, but the actual diagnosis of this child is very much in question.

Finally, *Intense Minds* is a collection of anecdotes and reminiscences about the suffering brought about by various symptoms of pediatric bipolar disorder (Anglada, 2006). The symptoms and the suffering are clearly portrayed, and the pain conveyed during the first-person accounts is vivid. Unfortunately, there is no evidence to suggest that the children have pediatric bipolar disorder. The symptoms are described in isolation by different children and with no pattern suggesting bipolar disorder. One chapter talks about anger; another talks about hypersexuality. Symptoms such as these, in isolation, are not sufficient for a diagnosis of bipolar disorder.

Weekly news magazines played an important role in supporting and disseminating the diagnosis of bipolar disorder in children. Highly influential was the August 19, 2002, issue of *Time* magazine in which bipolar disorder in childhood was the cover story (Kluger et al., 2002). It provided clinical descriptions of a nine-year-old and an adolescent both diagnosed with bipolar disorder. The nine-year-old did not seem to have the diagnosis; the adolescent did. Although the article notes in passing that the diagnosis is controversial, the overall tenor was very supportive of the diagnosis in children.

The scientific value of such articles is in good part determined by the quality of the experts the journalists elect to interview. Understandably, one of the sources for the article was Dr. Papalos, a pediatric bipolar expert of the day. Dr. Papalos informed the many readers of *Time* that pediatric bipolar disorder was like a tumor that had to be treated immediately or it would become much worse with time. He also noted without evidence that pediatric bipolar disorder is worse in the morning but often subsides in the afternoon. The article discusses the genetic basis of the disorder. The article does not consider the possibility that the disorder has increased because it is excessively diagnosed. The article concludes optimistically that many new drugs are currently in the process of being tested for the treatment of the disorder.

The May 26, 2008, edition of *Newsweek* ran a cover story on pediatric bipolar disorder. The article was almost entirely devoted to the case history of "Max," who was 10 years old at the time of the article and 2 years old at the time the diagnosis was first made (Carmichael, 2008). The article endorses Max's diagnosis of bipolar disorder. Max's main symptom seemed to be aggression that was severe, frequent, and unprovoked. The aggression began in his earliest toddler years and persisted with marginal improvement. Over his short life he had been on 38 different psychotropic medications. He did not respond well to them and developed a wide array of symptoms for which the medicines were blamed. At times he abruptly became depressed and suicidal but recovered in a matter of hours. Although Max is clearly a seriously disturbed child, there is no evidence that he meets *DSM-IV* criteria for bipolar disorder. Believing that he had bipolar disorder does not seem to have improved his symptoms.

The Sunday *New York Times Magazine* ran an article on September 14, 2008, that provided several case histories combined with the authors' observations of the children and families (Egan, 2008). This material provides a compelling impression of the appearance and behavior of children diagnosed as having pediatric bipolar disorder. The article seems to support the diagnosis of pediatric bipolar disorder for all of the cases. As in the other magazine articles discussed, the children are extremely aggressive and often dangerously out of control. After years of medication, psychotherapy, and special education efforts, the children remained impaired by their aggression and inability to conform to social expectations. A number of leaders in the field of bipolar disorder were interviewed for the article, and their comments supporting the diagnosis were reported at some length. Gabrielle Carlson, MD, presented the only dissenting view. Her comments were briefly reported and largely lost in the piece.

All of the articles make the obligatory comment that the diagnosis is controversial but do not develop the objections to the diagnosis substantially. The overall impression given to the reader is that the disorder exists and that the finest minds in child psychiatry are studying it. Reading the three articles at one sitting makes clear that these children do poorly with the treatments they have been provided. Their aggression continues, their families are devastated, their social skills are rudimentary, and their academic performance is limited. For the child patients described in these magazine articles, the diagnosis of bipolar disorder and the treatment based on this diagnosis have not been helpful.

These media presentations gained unusual force with the apparent endorsement of the disorder at the highest levels of the mental health scientific establishment—the National Institute of Mental Health (NIMH). Science is a major influence in the culture of mental health, and the National Institute of Mental Health is the most powerful force in the science of mental health in the United States. For decades, the best research in child and adult psychiatry in America has been performed at NIMH or funded by NIMH at universities around the country.

According to the article "What's Normal?" by the distinguished physician and *New Yorker* columnist Jerome Groopman, MD, an odd interaction occurred when *The Bipolar Child* crossed paths with the austere world of science at the National Institute of Mental Health (Groopman, 2007). In the article, Steve Hyman, MD, the former director of NIMH, described visits from parents of bipolar children, all of them clutching the book *The Bipolar Child* when discussing their children. These parents enthusiastically endorsed the book and the diagnosis of bipolar disorder in children. In the early 2000s the National Institute of Mental Health undertook a major research initiative for the study of pediatric bipolar disorder that would influence how the disorder was viewed by the child psychiatric community.

PROFESSIONAL SUPPORT FOR THE DIAGNOSIS

In April 2000, during the time of Dr. Hyman's directorship, NIMH convened a conference of researchers in pediatric bipolar disorder, many of whom had been funded by NIMH. The results of the conference were published in the *Journal of the American Academy of Child and Adolescent Psychiatry* under the title "National Institute of Mental Health Research Roundtable on Pre-pubertal Bipolar Disorder" (Nottelman, 2001). The article provided information to the practicing child psychiatry community about NIMH's thinking and plans for the study of the disorder. It also conveyed some of the thinking of leading child psychiatry researchers.

The article supported many research tactics for the study of pediatric bipolar disorder that are strongly criticized in this book. For example the "roundtable" seemed to endorse asking adult bipolar patients at what age their symptoms of bipolar disorder began in order to understand the age at which bipolar disorder might begin. The reported "data" are subject to all of the distortions of memory of long ago events reported by distressed patients. The Childhood Behavior Checklist (CBCL) was recommended as an important instrument in the study of pediatric bipolar disorder, although it was not designed with this purpose in mind and does not reflect *DSM-IV* criteria. Most important, the roundtable article incorrectly noted that prepubertal children met *DSM-IV* criteria for bipolar disorder and bipolar II disorder. It also recommended that children who did not meet all of the criteria, such as those described by Dr. Biederman, should be diagnosed as bipolar disorder NOS. It was suggested that the latter group *may have* (italics in the original article) bipolar disorder. The further study of bipolar disorder in preschool children was recommended. Overall, NIMH appeared to endorse a number of controversial propositions that had a major influence on clinical care and research for the next decade.

It is highly unusual for an NIMH roundtable discussion to be published in the *Journal of the American Academy of Child and Adolescent Psychiatry*—there are no other such articles of which I am aware. Although publication of the discussion seems to be an entirely reasonable and constructive activity from the perspective of NIMH and the *Journal*, it may have led to some unintended consequences. The *Journal* publishes primarily research articles, but it is read mostly by practicing child psychiatrists. It seems inevitable that the research issues discussed in the roundtable article eventually would be applied to the clinical care of patients. It is easy to see how a clinician might interpret the article as an indication that pediatric bipolar disorder is accepted as a diagnosis by NIMH, suggesting that it was now reasonable to identify and treat such patients in practice. The article is carefully and tentatively written, but for the busy reader it might have seemed that NIMH had given its support to the disorder's existence.

Following publication of the article, NIMH developed funded initiatives for research programs and invited university researchers to apply for grant money to study pediatric bipolar disorder.

NIMH's research support for the study of the disorder continued despite the publication of a well-reasoned critique of the disorder in a written heated debate between Rachel Gittleman-Klein, PhD, a distinguished researcher in the psychopathology of childhood, and Dr. Biederman (Biederman, Klein, Pine, & Klein, 1998). In the debate, Dr. Gittleman-Klein spelled out many of the reasons that pediatric bipolar disorder did not meet *DSM-IV* criteria for bipolar disorder. It seemed to me that Dr. Gittleman-Klein had won the debate, but NIMH was undeterred from providing research support for the disorder.

It is difficult to overestimate the sway that NIMH holds over psychiatry. Obtaining a NIMH research grant is a major "ticket punch" to a career at a university medical school. Those psychiatrists who work at university centers will invest hundreds of hours in efforts to obtain such a grant. To learn that there was a new area for funding undoubtedly led to intense activity among university psychiatrists and created in a twinkling stakeholders in the idea of childhood bipolar disorder. In general, if you receive money to study a particular area, you begin to find the area of increasing interest and importance. There is a natural inclination to be an advocate for the area in which you are working and funded.

NIMH, and university child psychiatrists funded by NIMH, have great influence on the field of child psychiatry and have been powerful forces in the spread of the concept of the bipolar child. Grant recipients wrote and published scientific papers on the disorder and its treatment. Many also frequently gave talks at professional meetings. Each paper they published and each talk they gave served, to some degree, to secure the illusion of the reality of the diagnosis in the professionals' minds. The specific content of each scientific paper was less important than the subtext or buried message of all of the papers, which was, "Not only does pediatric bipolar disorder exist, but as a measure of its importance, I am spending my valuable university time and NIMH money to do research on it." This helped create the illusion of a scientific foundation for the disorder that implicitly served to persuade professionals of its existence.

NIMH-funded university psychiatrists also tend to be "Key Opinion Leaders" ("KOLs" in the jargon of pharmaceutical companies) who exert a significant influence over how other child psychiatrists diagnose and prescribe. Psychiatrists in the community at times feel uncertain about the best way to proceed with a difficult case. Amid these uncertainties, the well-intentioned child psychiatrist often looks to the guidance of the Key Opinion Leaders in the field. These clinicians sometimes base their treatment on what they have heard from a KOL in the belief that if they do what the KOL does they are providing the best diagnosis and treatment currently available.

The NIMH funding, and consequent activities at scientific meetings and in professional journals, began to create an incessant drumbeat selling the diagnosis. Frequently, practicing psychiatrists were scolded in professional articles for underdiagnosing pediatric bipolar disorder. Although there was little scientific evidence that pediatric bipolar disorder existed, its presence seemed assured by the marketplace. Mental health consumers had embraced the diagnosis, as had the vast majority of mental health practitioners, and the psychiatric research establishment studying the disorder never seemed to miss an opportunity to advocate for it. What could not be gained in the science of the study of the disorder was easily achieved in the arena of public relations.

The pharmaceutical industry, always seeking out new markets, viewed the development of this new diagnosis with great interest. Drug companies recognize the invaluable influence (and marketing potential) of Key Opinion Leaders and court them assiduously. They offer lucrative opportunities to act as paid consultants, serve on advisory boards, and give talks to other doctors. It was through these pharmaceutical-company-sponsored talks that many child psychiatrists received instruction in the diagnosis of pediatric bipolar disorder. The talks were sponsored by companies that made drugs approved for use only in adults with bipolar disorder in the hopes that child psychiatrists would make the association and then use those drugs for children. The strategy seemed to work quite well. Although pharmaceutical companies are not allowed to advertise that a drug works or is safe in an age group or disease not specifically approved by the FDA, doctors are allowed to use drugs "off label" for any age or condition so long as the drug is on the market.

Aside from all of the external influences on physician behavior, there seems to be something about the diagnosis of pediatric bipolar disorder that is inherently appealing to the treating physician. Perhaps it is the complexity of the disorder, or it may be the complexity of using a combination of medications that until now had played almost no role in child psychiatry. The simplicity of the diagnosis of ADHD and its ease of treatment may have led to a degree of tedium for the office-based practitioner of child psychiatry. Pediatric bipolar disorder, in contrast, suggested some nuanced constellation of symptoms requiring a highly specialized pharmacologic skill set with drugs that were new to the child psychiatric community.

Parents of patients may be partly responsible as well. Many parents I see believe ADHD to be a commonplace and even stigmatizing diagnosis. They prefer, instead, to conceptualize their children as having bipolar disorder, which for many parents has come to be associated with creativity and intelligence. The authors of *The Bipolar Child* encourage this view when they write that many bipolar children "are extremely precocious and bright—doing everything early and with gusto. They seem like magical children, their creativity can be astounding, and the parents speak about them with real respect, and sometimes even awe" (Papolos & Papolos, 2006, p. 8).

In reality, given the choice of receiving a diagnosis of ADHD or one of bipolar disorder, ADHD is preferable. It is well understood and is easily and safely treated. In contrast, pediatric bipolar disorder is controversial, poorly understood, usually has a limited response to treatment, and has a well-known poor outcome (Geller & Luby, 1997; Strober et al., 1995).

PSYCHOLOGICAL CONSEQUENCES OF MISDIAGNOSIS

When a child is misdiagnosed with pediatric bipolar disorder, there are a number of negative consequences. The child may be given dangerous adult medications, often in combination, with long-term effects on children that are unknown. Also, the serious difficulties these children do have—such as ADHD and ODD—are often left untreated. The long-term psychological effects of misdiagnosis can also be considerable. It is useful to look to social science to understand some of the possible consequences of imposing the pediatric bipolar disorder diagnosis.

In the physical world, simply predicting the return of Halley's Comet or predicting the amount of snowfall for the coming winter will not change the course of Halley's Comet or the amount of snow that will fall. The situation is very different in predicting human behavior. Informing subjects, patients, or others about your prediction can change their behavior and the outcome of the prediction.

Psychiatry, and especially child psychiatry, is entangled with making predictions about human behavior. In the language of medicine the prediction is usually expressed as a prognosis, which is an estimate of the long-term outcome of the illness. The prognosis provides information about whether the illness will improve, get worse, be cured, or become chronic. In child psychiatry the process is even more complex, as predictions made about the outcome of an illness may serve as forecasts about the future functioning of the child as an adult.

In their seminal book *Pygmalian in the Classroom*, Robert Rosenthal, PhD, and Lenore Jacobson, EdD, considered at length situations in which a prediction has an influence on the phenomenon under study (Rosenthal & Jacobson, 1968, 1992). These authors explained that a prediction changes outcome. When applied to a person making a prediction about another person, such as a doctor making a prediction about a patient, a prediction is an expectation on the part of the person making it, and the expectation, which is then communicated to the patient, changes the patient. In that sense, just making the prediction may change behavior so that the prediction comes true. When a prediction (prophesy) changes the outcome of events so that the prediction comes true, it is called a "self-fulfilling prophesy."

Rosenthal and Jacobson cited extremely interesting studies that show how a person's expectation can change behavior—even of nonhumans. In one typical study, psychology students were each assigned a rat that would be observed in several learning tasks. The students were told (deceived, actually) that certain rats were brighter than others when, in reality, all of the rats had the same ability. The students were then asked to observe the speed at which their rats mastered certain basic tasks like maze running. At the end of the study, the rats that had been labeled brighter actually learned these tasks faster than rats not labeled brighter. It was speculated that the students may have treated the rats labeled brighter differently—handled them more frequently, for example—and that this may have led them to perform better.

Rosenthal and Jacobson note that elementary school teachers intuitively make predictions to themselves at the beginning of the school year about which of their students will do well and which will do poorly. These intuitive predictions may be based on racial bias or social class biases that are determined by the appearance and behavior of the students. The teachers often have access to other information as well, such as the student's previous performance in earlier grades. All of these intuitive judgments come together to create expectations about each child's performance during the school year, and the teachers may treat children differently based on these expectations. For example, they may spend less time with students they expect to do less well and more time with students they expect to improve. As a result, the children whom they view pessimistically may actually do less well simply because the teacher believed they would, and the teacher will have unwittingly created a self-fulfilling prophesy.

In an attempt to understand this phenomenon, Rosenthal and Jacobson studied the effect of teachers' expectations on academic performance, IQ, and student behavior. The study took place at an elementary school located in a working class community. The school divided students according to their ability, and there were three tracks in each grade: high, middle, and low. At the beginning of the school year an IQ test was administered to all of the children at the school. As part of the experiment, the teachers were deceived into believing that the IQ test served to identify those students who might be expected to have a "surge" in academic competence in the coming school year. This deception was part of the experiment. The names of 20% of the students in the school were selected, completely by chance, as those who would have a surge, and the names were given to their teachers. If the self-fulfilling prophesy were true, those students whom the teachers believed would surge would actually show improvements simply because of the teachers' expectations.

The experiment worked. There was a marked increase in IQ, grades, and behavior for the children identified as likely to surge. This was significantly greater than the improvement shown by the children not so identified. The study provides evidence that a change in expectations can lead to actual major changes in behavior and can even lead to changes in things previously thought to be relatively unchangeable, such as IQ.

What is the result of creating an expectation that a child has bipolar disorder? Diagnosing a child with a psychiatric illness he or she does not have creates fertile soil for a self-fulfilling prophecy. The child patient may begin to see himself or herself in a different light, as may the parents, teachers, siblings, and peers of the child (as well as a wide variety of other people with whom the child interacts). Cultural depictions of bipolar disorder or knowledge of adults who have the disorder will undoubtedly influence or affect how the child is viewed and how the child is expected to behave.

The role of self-fulfilling prophecy seems as if it has great potential for consideration in longitudinal studies of pediatric bipolar disorder. It is regrettable that it is never even mentioned as an idea in all of the published studies. For example, a large NIMH study from three university medical centers examined 263 children and adolescents with so-called bipolar spectrum disorders (Birmaher et al., 2006). The concept of the study was to follow these children for several years to learn what happened to their symptoms and whether they would develop into adult bipolar disorder patients with the classical *DSM-IV* appearance of bipolar disorder. As part of a longer-term longitudinal study, patients with an average age of 13 years were followed for two years and seen for evaluation every nine months. At the end of the two-year period the study found that 20% of the youth with bipolar II disorder—those with a less severe form of mania—met criteria for bipolar I disorder and 25% of those diagnosed with bipolar disorder NOS met criteria for either bipolar II disorder or bipolar I disorder. In other words, the children's disorders tended to became more typical of adult bipolar disorders over the two years.

It is easy to imagine that there was a strong expectation for the patients' bipolar symptoms to become more similar to adult versions of the disorder by the conclusion of the study. The research project team would have discussed this possible outcome with the child and the family, and it may have been a topic of conversation within the family as well. Yet the obvious role of the self-fulfilling prophecy is not mentioned in the article reporting the study. Given the vagaries of psychiatric illness and diagnosis and the influence of expectations on behavior, an omission of this obvious consideration is an important scientific issue.

From the perspective of patients and the psychiatrists who see them, the most disturbing implication of the self-fulfilling prophecy is the possibility of creating the illness in someone who might not otherwise have had it. Families can spend a good portion of their lives supporting the prophecy based on their own (mis)understanding of bipolar disorder and the limited evidence on which the prophecy is based. The effect this may have on a young child might take a novelist or a film-maker to portray fully.

CONCLUSION

The shrill marketing of pediatric bipolar disorder by the commercial media, along with support for the study of the disorder from NIMH and Key Opinion Leaders, threatened to overwhelm the dispassionate scientific consideration of the existence of the disorder and the possible risks involved in its diagnosis, treatment, and prevention. Publication of articles in the most prestigious psychiatric scientific journals lent incalculable authority to the unwarranted professional belief that the disorder existed and had been subjected to the most careful scrutiny.

It is reasonable to imagine or hope that science and its methods would balance the marketing and commercial pressures applied in selling the disorder. Yet for more than 15 years this did not seem to be happening. Instead, the interests and power of the pediatric bipolar community seemed to become increasingly entrenched. Evidence counter to the existence of the disorder was largely ignored—in fact there did not seem to be any evidence that might dislodge the proponents of the disorder from their beliefs—and acceptance of the existence of the disorder became impervious to argument. Although there were exceptions, until very recently, most protests took the form of quiet muttering between attendees after scientific meetings.

There were a few critics in American child psychiatry who challenged the establishment on this issue. Among early public critics were Drs. Rachel Gittleman-Klein (Biederman et al., 1998), Jon McClellan (McClellan, 2005), and David Shaffer, MD, the chief of the Division of Child Psychiatry at Columbia University College of Physicians and Surgeons. Dr. Shaffer was featured criticizing the pediatric bipolar disorder diagnosis in an episode titled "The Medicated Child" on the widely seen PBS program *Frontline* (Gaviria, 2008). His viewpoint will be especially influential in the future, as Dr. Shaffer is a prominent member of the child and adolescent section of the *DSM-V* task force. Sharna Olfman, PhD, recently edited *Bipolar Children,* a book critical of the disorder (Olfman, 2007). Critics outside of the United States such as David Healy, MD, from Wales, Anne Duffy, MD, FRCPC, from Canada, Peter Parry, MD, and Stephen Allison, MD, from Australia, and Richard Harrington, MD, and Tessa Myatt, MD, of the United Kingdom have made the case that the disorder was largely nonexistent in childhood (Duffy, 2007; Harrington & Myatt, 2003; Healy & Noury, 2007; Parry & Allison, 2008).

Currently there does seem to be a cultural and scientific shift away from the diagnosis. The *DSM-V* committee will have a major effect on the fate of the diagnosis.

REFERENCES

American Psychiatric Association. (2000). *Diagnostic and Statistical Manual of Mental Disorders* (4th ed. Text Revision ed.). Washington, DC: American Psychiatric Association.

Anglada, T. (2006). *Intense Minds: Through the Eyes of Young People with Bipolar Disorder.* Victoria BC, Canada: Trafford.

Anglada, T., Taylor, J., illustrator, & Ferguson, T., illustrator. (2004). *Brandon and the Bipolar Bear? A Story for Children with Bipolar Disorder.* Victoria BC, Canada: Trafford.

Biederman, J., Klein, R. G., Pine, D. S., & Klein, D. F. (1998). Resolved: Mania is mistaken for ADHD in prepubertal children. *J Am Acad Child Adolesc Psychiatry, 37*(10), 1091–1096; discussion 1096–1099.

Birmaher, B., Axelson, D., Strober, M., Gill, M. K., Valeri, S., Chiappetta, L., et al. (2006). Clinical course of children and adolescents with bipolar spectrum disorders. *Arch Gen Psychiatry, 63*(2), 175–183.

Carmichael, M. (2008, May 2008). Growing Up Bipolar: Max's World. *Newsweek.*

Duffy, A. (2007). Does bipolar disorder exist in children? A selected review. *Can J Psychiatry, 52*(7), 409–417.

Egan, J. (2008, September 12). The Bipolar Puzzle. *The New York Times Magazine.*

Faedda, G. L., & Austin, N. B. (2006). *Parenting a Bipolar Child: What to Do and Why.* Oakland, CA: New Harbinger Publications, Inc.

Gaviria, M. (Writer). (2008). The Medicated Child: WGBH Educational Foundation.

Geller, B., & Luby, J. (1997). Child and adolescent bipolar disorder: A review of the past 10 years. *J Am Acad Child Adolesc Psychiatry, 36*(9), 1168–1176.

Groopman, J. (2007, April 9). What's Normal? The difficulty of diagnosing bipolar disorder in children. *New Yorker, 83.*

Harrington, R., & Myatt, T. (2003). Is preadolescent mania the same condition as adult mania? A British perspective. *Biol Psychiatry, 53*(11), 961–969.

Healy, D. (2008). *Mania: A Short History of Bipolar Disorder.* Baltimore: Johns Hopkins University Press.

Healy, D., & Noury, J. L. (2007). Pediatric bipolar: An object of study in the creation of an illness. *International Journal of Risk & Safety in Medicine, 19*, 209–221.

Hebert, B., Hannah, J., illustrator, & Hebert, M., illustrator. (2005). *My Bipolar Roller Coaster Feelings Book.* Victoria BC, Canada: Trafford.

Kluger, J., Song Sora, D. C., Ressner, J., DeQuine, J., Sattley, M., Scalet, C., & Sieger, M. (2002). Manic depression: Young and bipolar. *Time.*

Lederman, J., & Fink, C. (2003). *The Ups and Downs of Raising a Bipolar Child: A Survival Guide for Parents.* New York: Fireside.

Loftus, E. F., & J.E., P. (1995). The formation of false memories. *Psychiatric Annals 25*, 720–725.

Lombardo, G. T. (2006). *Understanding the Mind of your Bipolar Child: The Complete Guide to the Development, Treatment, and Parenting of Children with Bipolar Disorder.* New York: St. Martin's Press.

McClellan, J. (2005). Commentary: Treatment guidelines for child and adolescent bipolar disorder. *J Am Acad Child Adolesc Psychiatry, 44*(3), 236–239.

Moynihan, R., & Henry, D. (2006). The fight against disease mongering: Generating knowledge for action. *PLoS Med, 3.*

Nottelman, E. (2001). National Institute of Mental Health research roundtable on prepubertal bipolar disorder. *J Am Acad Child Adolesc Psychiatry, 40*(8), 871–878.

Olfman, S. (Ed.). (2007). *Bipolar Children.* Westport, CT, and London: Praeger.

Papolos, D., & Papolos, J. (2006). *The Bipolar Child* (3rd ed.). New York: Broadway Books.

Parry, P., & Allison, S. (2008). Pre-pubertal paediatric bipolar disorder: A controversy from America. *Australas Psychiatry, 16*(2), 80–84; discussion 85–86.

Rosenthal, R., & Jacobson, L. (1968, 1992). *Pygmalion in the Classroom: Teacher Expectation and Pupils Intellectual Development.* Bethel, CT: Crown House Publishing, Irvington Publishers, Holt, Rinehart and Winston, Inc.

Strober, M., Schmidt-Lackner, S., Freeman, R., Bower, S., Lampert, C., & DeAntonio, M. (1995). Recovery and relapse in adolescents with bipolar affective illness: A five-year naturalistic, prospective follow-up. *J Am Acad Child Adolesc Psychiatry, 34*(6), 724–731.

Theisen, D., & Theisen, A. (2008). *Bipolar Bubbles: A Positive Journey Through the Eyes of a Child with Bipolar Disorder.* Indianapolis: Dog Ear Publishing.

Watters, E. (2010a, January 8). The Americanization of mental illness. *New York Times Magazine.*

Watters, E. (2010b). *Crazy Like Us: The Globalization of the American Psyche.* New York: Free Press.

Yan, J. (2010). DSM-5 postponed until 2013; Field trials scheduled for summer. *Psychiatric News, 45*, 2.

5

Child and Adolescent Depression: A Brief Introduction

Arguably, child psychiatry's most substantial contribution over the past 30 years has been in understanding childhood depression. The development of the contemporary concept of child depression was a lever to free child psychiatry from tradition-encrusted psychoanalytic clinical thinking and prescientific psychoanalytic methods of research, allowing the field to embrace contemporary modes of scientific study of childhood disorders. The new areas of study included biological psychiatry, psychopharmacology, and interest in the scientific assessment of childhood psychopathology. The study of childhood depression served to bring these trends together and apply them to this poorly understood clinical phenomenon.

Until the mid-1970s it was believed that depression did not exist in children below the age of 13. The myth of the happy childhood was a widely shared belief. There was nothing for children to fret about: sexually innocent, free from economic responsibility, and reared in loving families, the specter of a child feeling sad, hopeless, and suicidal was not in accord with the *Leave It to Beaver, Father Knows Best* television portrayals of American family life of the 1950s and 1960s.

Of course, child psychiatrists were keenly aware that childhood was a difficult struggle for their patients. Although child psychiatrists of that era were sophisticated about a number of aspects of childhood, most were blind to the phenomenon of childhood depression. Depression was felt to be too painful for children to tolerate. If a child were depressed, it was believed, the child would immediately flee the experience psychologically and translate the depressed feeling into another more bearable feeling, such as anger. This concept grew out of play therapy, the dominant treatment modality of the time. In play therapy, the child tells a story as he or she plays with a toy or draws a picture until a point is reached when the story and play create some anxiety in the child. At the moment the story and play create anxiety in the child, the child switches the play and stops the story. The child may choose a different activity or change the story that is told to avoid the anxiety the play has created. The child is often not aware of the anxiety, but to the play therapist it becomes clearly visible over the course of the play session.

Depression was felt to be similar to the anxiety-driven disruptions of play therapy. The child would not experience the depression directly but would move on quickly to other activities to avoid the painful feeling. With play therapy, the depression might slowly emerge to enable the child and therapist to discuss it. Initially the depression was not asked about directly.

This view of depression was closely related to another concept in the field at the time: masked depression. Masked depression in children and adolescents was depression concealed by the mask of other behaviors, such as silliness or aggression, to hide the underlying depression at the center of their difficulties. Behind these behaviors was the more fundamental depression that the therapist assumed to be present.

DIAGNOSING DEPRESSION IN CHILDREN AND ADOLESCENTS

The contemporary approach to treating childhood depression had many predecessors, but the flag-bearer for the revolution was Joachim Puig-Antich, MD, who was instrumental in developing the concept that children had depression and could meet *DSM* criteria for it. I vividly remember my own shock at seeing Dr. Puig-Antich's videos of depressed early elementary school aged children with drawn faces complaining of guilt, suicidality, and painful sadness much as a 60-year-old depressed adult might.

Dr. Puig-Antich and his colleagues developed one of the first semistructured clinical interviews to assess childhood psychopathology, the K-SADS (children's "kiddie" schedule for affective disorders and schizophrenia). It was based on a semistructured interview for adults, the SADS, and covered the entire spectrum of psychopathology in children and adolescents. The parent and the child were interviewed separately, and the interviewer had to weigh the response of both and arrive at what was regarded as the interviewer's best estimate of the severity of the symptom. At the end of each section of the interview the symptoms were used to calculate the *DSM* diagnosis.

The K-SADS interview was ground-breaking; it smashed the prohibition against asking children directly about symptoms of depression, anxiety, and suicidality. The child could and should be asked directly about symptoms of psychopathology, as children were more than capable of providing reasonable answers to the questions. It gave the interviewer the responsibility of assessing the patient's and parents' report and interpreting the responses to arrive at a score for the severity of the symptom. The interview further established support for the notion that the diagnosis of childhood disorders could be made using the same diagnostic criteria used in adults. The interviewer used *DSM* criteria developed for adults to arrive at the diagnosis at the conclusion of the K-SADS.

Dr. Puig-Antich was also an early investigator of antidepressants in children, the role of sleep in depressed children and adolescents, and the role of growth hormone in depressed children and adolescents. There was little precedent for the study of biological bases of psychopathology in childhood. His studies of childhood depression led the way into a new era of understanding and researching serious psychiatric disorders in childhood (Ryan, 2003).

Dr. Puig-Antich died suddenly and unexpectedly from an asthma attack on December 2, 1989, at the young age of 45 years. His independent research career had spanned only 12 years. Who would be the next Joachim Puig-Antich? Perhaps the efforts to answer this question fueled an overly zealous search to find bipolar disorder in children.

THE DIAGNOSIS OF DEPRESSION IN CHILDREN AND ADOLESCENTS AND *DSM-IV* CRITERIA

Dr. Puig-Antich's research effectively demonstrated that depression in childhood looks very much like depression in adulthood, and could be diagnosed using the same criteria. The *DSM- IV* criteria for major depression are listed in Table 5.1.

As shown, at least one of the first two symptoms must be present. The first symptom listed, depressed mood, includes a specific exception for children and adolescents: irritability may be substituted for depressed mood. This is one of the few places in *DSM-IV* where there is a specific recommendation for children and adolescents. Because almost all *DSM-IV* psychiatric diagnoses are associated with irritability, however, permitting irritability to substitute for depression has created difficulties in distinguishing depression from other psychiatric

TABLE 5.1. DSM-IV Criteria for Major Depressive Episode

A. Five (or more) of the following symptoms have been present during the same 2-week period and represent a change from previous functioning; at least one of the symptoms is either (1) depressed mood or (2) loss of interest or pleasure.

Note: Do not include symptoms that are clearly due to a general medical condition, or mood-incongruent delusions or hallucinations.

(1) depressed mood most of the day, nearly every day, as indicated by either subjective report (e.g., feels sad or empty) or observation made by others (e.g., appears tearful)

Note: In children and adolescents, can be irritable mood.

(2) markedly diminished interest or pleasure in all, or almost all, activities most of the day, nearly every day (as indicated by either subjective account or observation made by others)

(3) significant weight loss when not dieting or weight gain (e.g., a change of more than 5% of body weight in a month), or decrease or increase in appetite nearly every day

Note: In children, consider failure to make expected weight gains.

(4) insomnia or hypersomnia nearly every day

(5) psychomotor agitation or retardation nearly every day (observable by others, not merely subjective feelings of restlessness or being slowed down)

(6) fatigue or loss of energy nearly every day

(7) feelings of worthlessness or excessive or inappropriate guilt (which may be delusional) nearly every day (not merely self-reproach or guilt about being sick)

(8) diminished ability to think or concentrate, or indecisiveness, nearly every day (either by subjective account or as observed by others)

(9) recurrent thoughts of death (not just fear of dying), recurrent suicidal ideation without a specific plan, or a suicide attempt or a specific plan for committing suicide

B. The symptoms do not meet criteria for a Mixed Episode.

C. The symptoms cause clinically significant distress or impairment in social, occupational, or other important areas of functioning.

D. The symptoms are not due to the direct physiological effects of a substance (e.g., a drug of abuse, a medication) or a general medical condition (e.g., hypothyroidism).

E. The symptoms are not better accounted for by Bereavement, i.e., after the loss of a loved one, the symptoms persist for longer than 2 months or are characterized by marked functional impairment, morbid preoccupation with worthlessness, suicidal ideation, psychotic symptoms, or psychomotor retardation.

(Reprinted with permission from the *Diagnostic and Statistical Manual of Mental Disorders, Fourth Edition*, Text Revision [Copyright 2000]. American Psychiatric Association.)

illnesses of childhood. When irritability becomes a diagnostic criterion, it tends to create havoc in classification systems for children's
psychiatric illnesses.

The addition of irritability may be a hangover from the antiquated
concept of masked depression. Irritability may have been viewed as
masking depression in another era of child psychiatry, but it is a trans-
parent mask to a competent contemporary child psychiatrist. As
a famous child psychiatrist, Dennis Cantwell, MD, concisely noted,
"If there is a mask to depression in children and adolescents, it is a
thin mask" (American Academy of Child and Adolescent Psychiatry,
2007; Cantwell, 1983). By this he meant that to penetrate the mask,
little more is required than to ask the patient directly about the depressive symptoms.

The second *DSM-IV* symptom of depression is a loss of interest or
pleasure in daily activities. Although they may not admit to sad feelings, many depressed children and adolescents lose interest in or stop
doing previously enjoyed activities. They may stop athletic activities
or stop talking on the phone with friends. In general, a child who is not
depressed enjoys life. In depression, tasks and activities are experienced as joyless burdens.

Mark, for example, was a thin seven-year-old boy with learning disabilities who was doing poorly in school. His parents spent two to
three hours each night drilling him on his homework but were constantly disappointed by his poor performance on school tests of the
same material. They frequently complained, "He doesn't try." These
homework sessions quickly became tense and were suffused with an
atmosphere of criticism of Mark. The school was concerned about
Mark's poor academic performance and regularly sent notes home to
his parents about it. Over time Mark became withdrawn and refused
to leave the house when children in the neighborhood came to ask him
out to play.

In family therapy sessions Mark's soft voice became almost inau-
dible. He complained, "I hate myself and I hate my life." He scored in
the very depressed range on an inventory of depressive symptoms. As
part of his treatment I advised his parents to limit both their criticisms
of Mark and the amount of time they spent in homework sessions. I
reminded them of his diagnosis of learning disabilities and assured
them that he was trying. In addition to these measures I also placed
Mark on a medication for the treatment of depression.

His parents, both of whom had a history of depression themselves,
followed my instructions about limiting the homework. They also introduced a number of enjoyable activities for Mark and the family, such as

weekend visits to the zoo and other outings. Mark responded very well. He began to play with other children and seemed much happier, and his grades improved somewhat. Within a month of beginning treatment Mark asked to complete another inventory of depressive symptoms because he wanted to show me how much he had improved.

Inability to concentrate, as a symptom of depression, can be mistaken for ADHD. The difficulty in concentrating in depression has its onset with the onset of the depression. Symptoms of ADHD, in contrast, begin at a young age (before 7) and continue as the child ages.

Two percent of children aged 12 and below are estimated to have depression. The rates are much higher in adolescents—4–8%. The ratio of males to females suffering from depression changes with puberty as well. In elementary school aged children the ratio of males to females with depression is equal or 1:1. In adolescence the ratio changes and females with depression outnumber males with the same disorder in a ratio of 2:1. This sex ratio of depression persists throughout adulthood (American Academy of Child and Adolescent Psychiatry, 2007).

As in bipolar disorder, depression in children, adolescents, and adults is usually a recurrent disorder; it is characterized by relapses and remissions. The initial episode is self-limiting; the disorder will likely fade in one to eight months without treatment because of biological fluctuations within the individual. An absence of treatment can lead to tumultuous difficulties in the patient's life, including suicide. Twenty percent to 60% of children and adolescents have a recurrence in one to two years. Often the illness continues to recur throughout life.

Depression usually occurs in combination with other psychiatric disorders in children and adolescents. The most common disorders found along with depression are anxiety disorders, but ADHD, substance abuse, and delinquency can also be found. Depression in children and adolescents, as in adults, is a biological disorder that is in part genetic. Life events such as abuse, neglect, peer difficulties, and school failure can increase the likelihood of a depressive illness developing in those with a biological or genetic predisposition to the disorder.

As is true for all *DSM-IV* diagnoses, it is important to ascertain that the symptoms are not due to any underlying medical causes. Brain tumors or other brain ailments can lead to depression, as can difficulties with endocrine glands such as the thyroid gland and the adrenal gland. Some medications can cause depression, and all medications a child is taking should be reviewed by a physician to insure that none is associated with the possibility of depression. The stimulant medications for ADHD—a group of medications much discussed in this book—are associated with a condition closely resembling depression. I see this occasionally in my practice. A stimulant-medicated child may become socially withdrawn. The child may stop going out for recess at school and refuse to play with other children after school. Lowering the medication dose or switching to a different stimulant medication usually resolves the symptom quickly.

SUICIDE

Suicide is a constant threat in depression. Suicide attempts do occur in prepubertal children, but they are rare compared to the relatively high rates in adolescence. Surveys of children aged 10–14 years of age have been done. The suicide rate in this age range is 1.5 per 100,000, but most of the suicides occur in the 12–14-year age range. In contrast, the suicide rate is 8.2 per 100,000 in 15–19-year-olds (Gould, Greenberg, Velting, & Shaffer, 2003). Suicidality is strongly associated with both depression and bipolar disorder in adolescents. *Suicide threats regardless of age must always be taken very seriously and require immediate professional evaluation.* A false myth about suicide has been that those who talk about their suicidal feelings do not make suicide attempts. The opposite is true: those who talk to friends and family about suicidal wishes are at great risk for attempts to take their lives.

A closely related topic to depression and suicide is the role of antidepressants in the suicide of children, adolescents, and adults. In 2003, after a number of government hearings, the FDA concluded that antidepressants were associated with the onset of suicidal ideation in rare cases in children and adolescents. Although there were no suicide attempts or completed suicides in the children studied, antidepressants carry this FDA warning about their use. This concern remains controversial. Before the FDA warning in 2003 there had been a steady decline in the rates of completed suicide in children and adolescents that corresponded to the introduction in 1980 of a class of antidepressant medications called selective serotonin reuptake inhibitors ("SSRIs," among these the brand names Prozac, Zoloft, Paxil, and others). The FDA warnings were issued in 2003 and were accompanied by a 20% decline in the prescription of antidepressants. Associated with the decline in antidepressant prescriptions, the suicide rate in children and adolescents began to climb. In 2004 it had increased by 14% in the United States. An identical situation was reported from the Netherlands where antidepressant use had also decreased after the FDA warning. In the Netherlands, as the prescriptions of antidepressants declined the suicide rates increased dramatically. The evidence strongly suggests that the FDA warnings had the unintended consequence of increasing the suicide rates of children and adolescents (Gibbons et al., 2007). To address this controversy and other disputes about the use of antidepressants in children and adolescents is beyond the scope of this book.

DEPRESSION AND BIPOLAR DISORDER

Depression is an integral part of adult bipolar disorder, with the patient usually at some point in the bipolar illness cycling into a depression phase that may come to dominate the illness. The patient may cycle from depression to a normal state and then back to depression many times over his or her lifetime with only a single episode of mania. The manic episode in such a patient enables the clinician to diagnose bipolar disorder based on *DSM-IV* criteria and indicates to the clinician that the patient has bipolar disorder and not simply a depressive disorder. The knowledge that the patient has bipolar disorder influences the medication choice of the clinician.

CONCLUSION

Depression in childhood and adolescence is a major issue for child psychiatry and is of great concern for the general public. Some of the aspects of this important topic have been introduced because of their relationship to pediatric bipolar disorder. Depression can be diagnosed with relative ease in children and adolescents. It usually responds well to treatment. Because of the high risk of suicide associated with this disorder, immediate professional evaluation of symptoms of depression is necessary.

REFERENCES

American Academy of Child and Adolescent Psychiatry. (2007). Practice parameter for the assessment and treatment of children and adolescents with depressive disorders. *J Am Acad Child Adolesc Psychiatry, 46*(11), 1503–1526.

American Psychiatric Association. (2000). *Diagnostic and Statistical Manual of Mental Disorders* (4th ed. Text Revision ed.). Washington, DC: American Psychiatric Association.

Cantwell, D.P. (1983). Depression in childhood: Clinical picture and diagnostic criteria. In D.P. Cantwell & G. Carlson (Eds.), *Affective disorders in Childhood and Adolescence: An Update.* New York: Spectrum.

Gibbons, R.D., Brown, C.H., Hur, K., Marcus, S.M., Bhaumik, D.K., Erkens, J.A., et al. (2007). Early evidence on the effects of regulators' suicidality warnings on SSRI prescriptions and suicide in children and adolescents. *Am J Psychiatry, 164*(9), 1356–1363.

Gould, M.S., Greenberg, T., Velting, D.M., & Shaffer, D. (2003). Youth suicide risk and preventive interventions: A review of the past 10 years. *J Am Acad Child Adolesc Psychiatry, 42*(4), 386–405.

Ryan, N.D. (2003). The Joaquim Puig-Antich legacy. *J Child Adolesc Psychopharmacol, 13*(3), 223–226.

6

Did Romeo and Juliet Have Bipolar II Disorder? Bipolar Disorder in Adolescence

Although *DSM-IV* bipolar disorder exists in adolescents, it is overdiagnosed. Often, as was true with prepubertal children, adolescents who are aggressive are misdiagnosed as having bipolar disorder because of the severity of their aggression (Blader & Carlson, 2007). Also, because adolescence is a period of strong feelings and intense emotional states, certain aspects of normal adolescence can sometimes resemble symptoms of mania, contributing to misdiagnosis. This chapter will explore some of the concerns that are particular to diagnosing bipolar disorder in adolescents.

ROMEO AND JULIET

Reducing one of the greatest love stories in Western literature to the dry listing of symptoms of a psychiatric disorder risks mocking both Shakespeare and *DSM-IV*. Yet there is some reason for considering these distinctly separate world views together. Romantic love and sexuality become important in adolescence, and suicidality, rare before adolescence, greatly increases. Adolescence is a period of strong emotions, strong sexual urges, great ambitions, intense longings, and at times, despair, hopelessness, and suicidality. Recent research has found that the enthusiasms and feelings of many healthy adolescents have much in common with adult mania. This may offer one important explanation for the overdiagnosis of bipolar disorder in adolescence; many of the symptoms of mania are part of the normal developmental course of adolescence. This is particularly true for hypomania, a less severe form of mania found in the bipolar II disorder diagnosis. Though hypomania does not meet the *DSM-IV* criteria for mania, the symptoms of the two are nearly identical except the duration is less (four days rather than the seven required for mania), and the symptoms do not impair functioning. For the diagnosis of bipolar II disorder, a hypomanic episode is required along with a history of at least one major depressive episode.

In an especially interesting study, Serge Brandt, PhD, and colleagues in Basel, Switzerland, scientifically compared romantic love in adolescents to hypomania in adults (Brandt, Luethi, von Planta, Hatzinger, & Holsboer-Trachsler, 2007). The authors noted the many similarities: euphoria, elation, intense goal-directed activity, and elevated sexual arousal are some of the most obvious. The Brandt group studied two groups of normal adolescents who were and were not in love and compared them with adults diagnosed with hypomania. By their own reports, one group of 60 adolescents was in the early stage of intense romantic love. They reported they were "madly in love." This group was asked three modified questions from a questionnaire designed to measure obsessive-compulsive disorder: "How much time do you think of the other person?" "While thinking of the other person do you feel distracted?" and "How well can you resist the need to think of the other person?" Their answers were rated with a maximum combined score of 12 for the 3 questions. Those with a score of six and above were admitted to the group of early-stage intense romantic love. This group was compared to another group of 47 adolescents who were either not intensely in love or not in love at all. The adolescents were then compared to 186 adult outpatients diagnosed with bipolar II disorder.

All the participants were given a hypomania symptoms questionnaire that asked about symptoms such as thinking quickly, spending too much money, and heightened self-esteem. The adolescents who were intensely in love scored almost identically to the adult hypomanic patients who had bipolar II disorder. The adolescents who were not intensely in love (or not in love at all) scored much lower.

Next, because decreased need for sleep is often reported as part of mania and hypomania, the sleep of the adolescents who were intensely in love was compared to the sleep of the adolescents who were not intensely in love or not in love at all. Sleep diaries were used; each morning the adolescents wrote down many aspects of the previous night's sleep. The adolescents who were intensely in love slept less but felt better rested than the adolescents who were not intensively in love or not in love at all. The intensely in love group also felt they had had a better quality of sleep, were able to concentrate better when awake, and felt more relaxed. The study suggests that hypomania is a regularly encountered feature of adolescents in love. Rather than a sign of psychopathology, romantic love is a normal aspect of psychological development. Romantic states, frequent in adolescence, may contribute to an overestimate of the number of cases of bipolar disorder in adolescents.

Another study supports the ubiquity of manic symptoms in adolescence. Tijssen and colleagues in Maastricht, The Netherlands, used standardized symptom scales to interview 1,395 normal 14–17-year-olds at four time points over the course of more than eight years (Tijssen, van Os, Wittchen, Lieb, Beesdo, Mengelers, Krabbendam, et al., 2010). Almost 40% of the adolescents had at least one symptom of mania. As the Tijssen group notes, "(Hypo)manic symptoms may be conceived partially as pertaining to normal adolescent development" (Tijssen, van Os, Wittchen, Lieb, Beesdo, Mengelers, & Wichers, 2010, p. 296).

Establishing the finding that hypomanic symptoms are relatively common in adolescents is crucial in understanding the limited capacity of these symptoms to predict bipolar disorder. The more common a symptom is, the less helpful it is in predicting a relatively rare and specific psychiatric disorder such as bipolar disorder. For example, most people who develop pneumonia have an earlier symptom of a runny nose, but most people with a runny nose never develop pneumonia. The same may be true to a lesser degree for manic symptoms in adolescents. Simple presence of a common symptom may have no bearing on the eventual development of an uncommon disease.

There is a tendency to infer the existence of a disease based on the presence of a few symptoms. The categorical approach to diagnosis currently used in *DSM-IV* provides some protection from sliding too quickly from some symptoms of a diagnosis to the diagnosis itself. With the "dimensional approach" advocated by many, disorders are seen as existing on a spectrum of symptoms and symptom severity. Those who have some of the symptoms are on the spectrum of the disorder, and there is not a meaningful difference between those who have all of the criteria for the disorder and those who have some symptoms but not enough to meet the formal *DSM* criteria for the diagnosis. In pediatric bipolar disorder, in particular, it is important not to confuse those with some symptoms of the disorder with those who have the actual *DSM-IV* disorder.

AGGRESSION AND THE MISDIAGNOSIS OF BIPOLAR DISORDER IN AN ADOLESCENT

In addition to romantic love, sexuality, and the high frequency of hypomanic symptoms, aggressive symptoms are often misinterpreted as diagnostic of bipolar disorder. Adolescents who are aggressive are frequently misdiagnosed with bipolar disorder because of the severity of their aggression. This was the case with Joey, a 15-year-old who had been psychiatrically hospitalized. I was called in one Monday morning to consult about his case after he had acted as the ringleader of a "riot" on the unit over the weekend. The adolescent patients had refused to follow any of the directives of the weekend staff and had decided to run the unit themselves. As the regular staff returned to work on Monday morning they, along with the hospital security staff, were able to restore order to the unit, and all the patients except Joey participated in morning routines and began to attend school in the classroom on the unit. Joey had refused to acquiesce to the restoration of unit rules and kept violently insisting that he and the rest of the patients were going to remain in charge of the unit.

Joey was enraged. He was physically assaulting clinical staff members and was struggling with hospital security staff when I arrived. He was placed in restraints and required an injection of medication to calm him and to quiet what had become a dangerous confrontation. During the turmoil of the restraint procedure, based on the severity of his aggression, the head nurse began to exclaim loudly, "He's bipolar, he's bipolar!" The severity of his aggression had led her to believe that he had bipolar disorder. He had an almost lifelong history of aggressive behavior both at home and at school and had had frequent contacts with the law, including several arrests and truancy. His behavior was chronic, not episodic. He had no history of manic episodes. This scenario is not uncommon; aggressive adolescents are at risk for being diagnosed as having bipolar disorder.

BIPOLAR DISORDER IN AN ADOLESCENT

In contrast with prepubertal children, *DSM-IV* bipolar disorder does occur in adolescents. Although this chapter has emphasized how some symptoms in adolescents may lead to an unwarranted diagnosis of bipolar disorder, it is paramount for parents to understand the more pathological implications of manic symptoms in adolescents, particularly when these symptoms are clearly different from the adolescent's baseline behavior.

Jean is a typical case. She was a 16-year-old honors high school student with a love of rock music. She excelled at academic subjects, particularly math, but did not find school interesting. She liked going to rock concerts and watching music videos with her friends. In the middle of the school year she suddenly changed. Her interest in rock music became all-encompassing, and she talking incessantly of her desire to become a producer of music videos. She stopped attending most of her usual after-school activities and instead spent hours watching music videos, reading about them, and developing complicated plans to direct and produce them. Around this time she announced that she no longer needed more than an hour or two of sleep. She could be found at all hours alone in her bedroom feverishly working on music video designs in a state of great excitement. She decided that her (average) drawing ability was actually advanced, and she spent long hours drawing pictures she believed could be incorporated into music videos. During this unusual period, which lasted for six weeks, she also became active sexually with two different boys and experimented with drinking to excess. Neither sexual activity nor drinking was behavior Jean had engaged in prior to the episode. She refused help, and her parents and friends were quite concerned.

After about six weeks, Jean began to feel depressed. She became withdrawn and apathetic and refused to talk to her friends or family. She began sleeping long hours, and her personal hygiene deteriorated. She lost interest in her plans to become a music video producer. She fought with her parents and perceived their comments as slights and criticisms. Her symptoms worsened over the course of three weeks, and feeling trapped and hopeless, she began to think about killing herself. She believed that she would never feel better, and she wrote suicide notes to her friends and family. On the night before her planned suicide Jean went to a rock concert to say goodbye to the experience she had most loved. During the concert she became convinced that the performer was singing words of encouragement directly to her. Moved by the singer at this concert, she decided to give up her plan for suicide and asked to see a psychiatrist for help.

The psychiatrist recognized the likelihood of bipolar disorder and began her on a mood stabilizer. Her mood improved considerably. Over the next six months she enrolled in an arts college and studied music video making. She loved the school and made many friends who shared her interests in music. At this point she decided that the psychiatrist was wrong and that she did not have bipolar disorder. She felt that she no longer needed the psychiatrist and stopped taking her medication. She continued without medication or treatment for the next year. As a condition of continuing to pay for her tuition and board, her mother insisted that she return to the psychiatrist, which she did. The psychiatrist recommended medication to prevent another cycle of her bipolar disorder, but Jean steadfastly refused, believing herself to be free from the threat of future psychiatric difficulties.

As this case illustrates, bipolar disorder does occur in adolescents and looks similar to bipolar disorder in adults. Adolescents who exhibit manic symptoms should be evaluated by a psychiatrist. This is particularly urgent if there is a change in usual behavior. Failure to appreciate the nature of the diagnosis in an adolescent can lead to the illness becoming more and more severe until the adolescent becomes psychotic. Treatment earlier in the course of the illness may interrupt this process. Suicide, always a risk in adolescents, is a greatly increased risk in those adolescents diagnosed with bipolar disorder. Another scourge of adolescence, drug abuse, is markedly increased in adolescents with bipolar disorder. It is imperative for parents to arrange a professional evaluation for adolescents with manic symptoms.

CONCLUSION

In 1939, Anna Freud, a well-known pioneer in child psychoanalysis and daughter of Sigmund Freud, presented a view of adolescence as a period of tumultuous emotions and struggles against the strong forces of sex and aggression (Freud, 1968). She coined the phrase "adolescent turmoil" and viewed it as an expectable part of adolescence. Daniel Offer, MD, and colleagues, using more contemporary interview techniques, found in contrast to what Anna Freud might have predicted that most adolescents were content and pleased to follow their parents' rules (Offer, Marcus, & Offer, 1970). The findings of the Brandt group and the Tijssen group seem more aligned with the more volatile view of adolescence depicted by Anna Freud. Doubtless there are groups of adolescents to whom one or the other characterizations apply, or they may apply to the same adolescents at different times. Understanding the emotions and behaviors of adolescents is a complex task for their parents and the professionals who work with them.

REFERENCES

Blader, J.C., & Carlson, G.A. (2007). Increased rates of bipolar disorder diagnoses among U.S. child, adolescent, and adult inpatients, 1996–2004. *Biol Psychiatry, 62*(2), 107–114.

Brandt, S., Luethi, M., von Planta, A., Hatzinger, M., & Holsboer-Trachsler, E. (2007). Romantic love, hypomania, and sleep pattern in adolescents. *J Adolesc Health, 41*(1), 69–76.

Freud, A. (1968). *The Ego and the Mechanisms of Defence.* London: Hogarth Press and the Institute of Psychoanalysis.

Offer, D., Marcus, D., & Offer, J.L. (1970). A longitudinal study of normal adolescent boys. *Am J Psychiatry, 126*(7), 917–924.

Tijssen, M.J., van Os, J., Wittchen, H.U., Lieb, R., Beesdo, K., Mengelers, R., et al. (2010). Evidence that bipolar disorder is the poor outcome fraction of a common developmental phenotype: an 8-year cohort study in young people. *Psychol Med, 40*(2), 289–299.

Tijssen, M.J., van Os, J., Wittchen, H.U., Lieb, R., Beesdo, K., Mengelers, R., Krab-bendam, L. et al. (2010). Prediction of transition from common adolescent bipolar experiences to bipolar disorder: 10-year study. *Br J Psychiatry*, *196*(2), 102–108.

PART II

Medications and Pediatric Bipolar Disorder

Other topics will be briefly considered in this chapter, such as the use of these medications for the treatment of aggression in children and adolescents not diagnosed with bipolar disorder. The next chapter, "Clinical Trials," will consider how it is decided whether these drugs work in children and adolescents.

LITHIUM

Lithium is the drug most often associated with the successful treatment of adult bipolar disorder. As early as the 1890s lithium was used in health spas and tonic waters, a practice that died out by the early 1900s. Lithium was also briefly used as a salt substitute in the United States because it was believed that it did not lead to increased blood pressure as table salt does. Chemically, lithium is a salt; it looks and tastes like table salt. Shortly after lithium's introduction for this purpose, however, three people died and five became seriously ill, and in 1949 it was removed from the market (Georgotas & Gershon, 1981). By coincidence, just prior to its removal from the market as a food, its use as a potential treatment for bipolar disorder was under study. In 1949, John Cade, an Australian psychiatrist, was seeking to determine whether patients who were manic were chemically different from normal patients and whether he could identify the chemical difference. He found that when he injected the urine of patients with mania to guinea pigs it was more toxic than when he injected the urine of people who did not have mania. During his investigations, to concentrate the urine he injected the guinea pigs with a form of lithium and noted that the guinea pigs became calmer than they had been prior to the lithium. He then gave lithium to a series of human patients with mania who had been hospitalized for an extended period. Many quickly recovered and left the hospital, which led him to conclude that lithium was helpful in the treatment of manic patients (Mitchell & Hadzi-Pavlovic, 1999). Mogens Schou, a psychiatrist from Copenhagen, was one of the early investigators to appreciate that lithium not only reduced manic episodes in what was then called manic-depressive illness but that it also seemed to play a role in their prevention. He was also the first to note that it helped patients with recurrent depression (Rosenthal & Goodwin, 1982).

Although lithium eventually was sold and used as a psychiatric medication, there were several factors that seemed to have inhibited its widespread use. First was the cloud created by the deaths associated with its use as a salt substitute (Johnson & Gershon, 1999). Second, the very simplicity of lithium as an element found in nature seemed to argue against its having an effect on brain functioning in such a complex psychiatric illness as bipolar disorder. Finally, the pioneers in the development of the use of lithium for psychiatric illness lived in countries, such as Australia and Denmark, that were not at the centers of influence for the adoption of psychiatric treatments as were Great Britain and the United States. Lithium was not approved by the FDA until 1970, after Schou and his colleagues conducted exhaustive clinical trials to prove its effectiveness in the treatment of bipolar disorder in adults.

Currently, lithium is one of the best-studied and least-expensive agents for the treatment of the manic phase of bipolar disorder in adults. In general, it is as effective as any other agent used today. It has been found to be effective in adults with bipolar disorder in 5 double-blind placebo controlled studies, the most rigorous method of assessing how well a drug works, as well as 16 other studies that had less scientific rigor (Goodwin & Jamison, 2007a). Lithium has also been found in 10 double-blind trials to be useful in the treatment of the depressed phase of bipolar disorder in adults (Goodwin & Jamison, 2007b).

When it comes to the use of lithium in children, however, the results are not at all clear. Most studies have not been conducted with the same rigor as those conducted in adults, and most of the studies were not with children diagnosed with pediatric bipolar disorder. In three studies, lithium was found to be effective for aggression in psychiatrically hospitalized children and adolescents who were not diagnosed with bipolar disorder (Campbell et al., 1984; Campbell et al., 1995; Malone et al., 2000) but there are other studies, in other settings or other circumstances, that do not find lithium to be helpful in childhood or adolescent aggression (Carlson et al., 1992; Rifkin et al., 1997; Klein, 1991). Some researchers report that lithium alone may be effective for pediatric bipolar disorder, but at this point there is no consensus that this is the case. Three scientifically sound double-blind studies (see next chapter) have been reported. In one double-blind study, lithium was effective for the treatment of bipolar disorder in substance-abusing adolescents (Geller et al., 1998) but in two other double-blind studies of lithium alone in bipolar adolescents, lithium was not effective (Kafantaris et al., 2004; Kowatch et al., 2000). In children and adolescents lithium seems most effective when given in combination with another agent such valproate or risperidone (Findling et al., 2003; Findling et al., 2005; Findling et al., 2006; Pavuluri et al., 2004; Pavuluri et al., 2006). When lithium is given with another medication, the effect of lithium is more difficult to assess. A considerable amount of ambiguity surrounds the use of lithium in children and adolescents. These uncertainties have been recognized at a national level, and a major research study with federal funding has been launched to assess the effectiveness and best dosing strategies of lithium for children and adolescents diagnosed with bipolar disorder (Findling et al., 2008). Lithium is associated with a large number of side effects in children, adolescents, and adults. Although a psychiatrist and cooperative patient can work together to manage these side effects, lithium does require careful monitoring if it is to be used safely.

Because the dose of the medicine taken by mouth does not automatically lead to a correct blood level, blood must be drawn and tested periodically or it can rise to the point where it becomes lethal. In general, the blood level of lithium for an acute manic episode in adults is recommended to be between 0.8 and 1.2 millimoles per liter (mmol/L). If it gets to 2.0 in an adult it can begin to cause serious side effects. It is commonplace in lithium management that the therapeutic blood levels rise to close to lethal levels. Even innocuous events can quickly lead to toxic blood levels. The heat of summer can raise levels because of water loss from sweating. When levels rise there may be nausea, vomiting, and though rare, even seizures followed by death. An entire unit of a state psychiatric hospital for children, for example, had to be medically hospitalized for lithium toxicity one summer because the children's lithium levels rose dangerously during a heat wave. Toxic lithium blood levels can be reduced, but neurological damage sustained during lithium toxicity may rarely be irreversible. Memory difficulties and difficulties walking have been reported as irreversible side effects of lithium toxicity (Freeman, Wiegand, & Gelenberg, 2009).

Other serious side effects of lithium include damage to the kidneys, thyroid, brain, and sexual system. These problems occur in only a minority of patients but require monitoring.

There are many less serious side effects of lithium, such as hand tremors, weight gain, and acne, that are particularly disturbing to adolescents and young adults and can quickly lead to a patient refusing to take the medicine. As one male adolescent diagnosed with bipolar disorder who was taking lithium complained, "This girl I met could tell I was on lithium. She could see my hands shaking and saw my face was broken out. She said, 'You're on lithium; I can tell.' I said, 'No I'm not,' but she insisted, 'You are, I can tell.'" This upset him enough that he asked to be removed from the drug.

The many side effects associated with lithium can interfere with treatment and necessitate careful monitoring by a knowledgeable physician. Nonetheless, lithium remains an effective treatment for adult bipolar disorder. Estimates are that approximately 50% of adults with bipolar disorder will respond to the medication, and a knowledgeable physician can reduce most of the side effects. For an adult patient correctly diagnosed with bipolar disorder who responds to treatment, the personal discomfort of taking the drug might seem a modest cost for the incalculable benefit of treating the illness. There is no evidence that this is the case for children.

VALPROATE

Valproate (brand name Depakote) is an anticonvulsant that is representative of a large number of medications used to treat bipolar disorder in that it was originally used as a treatment for seizure disorders and was only later found to be effective in treating bipolar disorder. It was first discovered to have antiseizure properties by the French chemist Hélène Meunier and her colleagues in 1963 and began to be used to treat seizures in the United States in the late 1970s. It was approved by the FDA for the treatment of adult bipolar disorder in 1995 (Bowden & McElroy, 1995). There are other medications approved for the treatment of seizures that are often used to treat bipolar disorder. There are several different formulations of valproate on the market in the United States.

In general, the effect of valproate is comparable to that of lithium. In seven double-blind trials, valproate worked as well as lithium and better than a placebo for adult bipolar disorder (Bowden, 2009).

Valproate has been studied in the treatment of children diagnosed with bipolar disorder and children with aggression. There have been several "open-label" studies reporting that valproate is helpful in children diagnosed with bipolar disorder (Papatheodorou et al., 1995; West, Keck, & McElroy, 1994; Wagner et al., 2006). In open-label studies, in contrast to double-blind studies, the patients and doctors know that the patient is receiving the medication and therefore are susceptible to bias in reporting the medication effects. The knowledge of having received a drug has been shown, in and of itself, to improve symptoms. Open-label studies are not a rigorous way of testing a medication and are not accepted by the FDA.

There are a handful of double-blind studies of valproate in pediatric bipolar disorder. The results are contradictory and will be discussed in the next chapter. Also, there have been two double-blind studies showing that valproate can be helpful in aggressive adolescents (Donovan et al., 2000; Steiner, Saxena, & Chang, 2003).

Despite limited scientific evidence, the use of anticonvulsants for psychiatric illness in children and adolescents without seizures more than doubled from 1990 to 2000. This substantial increase is another source of concern about the overdiagnosis of pediatric bipolar disorder.

In 1990, anticonvulsants played a minor role in the treatment of child psychiatric illness. In a Tennessee Medicaid study dated 1992 only 11% of such medications prescribed for children aged birth to 18 years of age were used for patients to treat a psychiatric illness. Over the following decade this number more than doubled in that state (Cooper, Federspiel, Griffen, & Hickson, 1997). In 2000, the use of anticonvulsants in a Medicaid population of children 17 years of age and younger was examined in one mid-Atlantic state. Of the 4,522 child and adolescent patients taking anticonvulsants, 68% had a psychiatric diagnosis without a seizure disorder. Valproate was the most frequently prescribed anticonvulsant (Zito et al., 2006).

A different study by a large managed-care research scientist, Enid Hunkeler, and her colleagues supports and extends the findings of the Zito group. This study used data from Kaiser Permanente in Northern California, a large health maintenance organization (HMO) whose patients are more affluent than those studied by the Zito group. Diagnoses and medications of children aged 5 through 17 years were examined from 1995 to 2003. There was a 650% increase in the number of children receiving anticonvulsants for bipolar disorder from 1995 to 2003. In 1995 only 4.8% of children receiving anticonvulsants had a bipolar disorder diagnosis, and by 2003 that number had risen to 31.1% (Hunkeler, Fireman, & Lee, 2005).

The unexpected increase in the use of anticonvulsants for psychiatric problems in children and adolescents is surprising given the limited number of studies that support their effectiveness in those conditions in this age range. This is made more disturbing when one considers the significant side effects associated with their use.

When medical studies indicate that a drug carries serious or even fatal side effects, the FDA can require the pharmaceutical company to place a "black box warning" on the label of the drug or in the literature describing it. It is regarded as the FDA's strongest warning. The "black box warning" for valproate (brand name Depakote), a very commonly used agent for pediatric bipolar disorder, indicates that, although rare, taking the medication can lead to liver damage and fatal pancreatitis. Although not contained in the black box warning, weight gain is a major side effect of the medication, and the long-term jeopardy to the health of the patient created by excessive weight gain is more widely appreciated than it was in the past. Additional side effects include sleepiness, changes in blood cells, and shakiness. Baldness or hair thinning is another side effect.

Particularly disturbing is the tendency of valproate to be masculinizing to females, including increased body hair growth, the development of male hair patterns on the scalp, and menstrual irregularities. In addition, valproate is associated with the development of a medical gynecologic syndrome called polycystic ovary syndrome (PCOS), an illness characterized by the development of cysts on the ovary, obesity, and masculinization. A recent major NIMH study of bipolar disorder in adults, the STEP-BD study, found 7.5 times the rate of PCOS in women aged 18 to 45 taking valproate (10.5%) compared to those taking other anticonvulsants for bipolar disorder (1.4%) (Joffe et al., 2006). This raises a concern about the use of the medication in prepubertal girls, adolescent girls, and women of child-bearing age.

RISPERIDONE

Risperidone (brand name Risperdal) is representative of a large class of medications called antipsychotics. Antipsychotic medications were first used in adult patients with schizophrenia, a serious disorder characterized by delusions (deeply held beliefs that are not true), hallucinations (seeing or hearing things that are not present), and a wide array of other disabling symptoms. Chlorpromazine (brand name Thorazine), which began to be used in 1952, was the first antipsychotic medication to dramatically reduce the symptoms of schizophrenia. With the use of this medication thousands of patients confined to state hospitals for a lifetime improved to the point where they could be released. Almost all seemed to improve but continued to display significant disturbances. Although the hallucinations and delusions decreased, the patients still seemed self-preoccupied and withdrawn. In general, they had only marginal interest in the outside world or issues of the day; their interest in other people was minimal. All required continuing medication to maintain their improvement. The medication had many side effects.

Several other medications similar to chlorpromazine were developed in an effort to reduce more symptoms and have fewer side effects. These medications are now known as "first-generation anti-psychotics," or FGAs. All are approximately equal to chlorpromazine in reducing the symptoms of schizophrenia and differ mainly in terms of their side effects (Nasrallah & Tandon, 2009).

One group of side effects that is typical of FGAs, including chlorpromazine, is known as "extrapyramidal symptoms," or "EPS," because the symptoms in this group are involved with a part of the nervous system known as the "extrapyramidal tract." Some side effects are similar to the symptoms of Parkinson's disease: slowed walking, drooling, lack of facial expression, stiffness of limbs, and tremors. Another side effect is "akathisia," an extremely unpleasant sense of inner restlessness that causes patients to almost continuously move. For many of these side effects, medications can be given that reduce or eliminate the symptoms. Tardive dyskinesia is another side effect of FGAs. It includes a variety of involuntary movements such as tongue rolling, lip smacking, and jerky motions of the body. Of great concern, tardive dyskinesia is potentially irreversible even if the medication is stopped (Dursun, Haddad, & Barnes, 2004).

Clozapine (brand name Clozaril), an antipsychotic medication developed in the early 1960s, was remarkable for decreasing the rates of EPS side effects. These lower rates initially disguised its potential for successfully treating schizophrenia, as many psychiatrists and psychopharmacologists at that time believed that the development of EPS was linked to the antipsychotic's effectiveness. Because clozapine did not seem to cause EPS, it was felt that it could not be effective for schizophrenia. With further study, however, it became clear that clozapine was exceptionally effective in the reduction of schizophrenia symptoms and it began to be used to treat schizophrenic patients who had not responded to FGAs. Clozapine came to be known as the first second-generation antipsychotic (SGA) (Marder & Wirshing, 2009).

Regrettably, clozapine had a number of new side effects. In particular, in some cases it suddenly and dramatically reduced the white blood cells in the body to zero or to extremely low levels. Several patients died. This greatly inhibited the widespread adoption of clozapine as a treatment for schizophrenia. The medication continues to be used to this day for schizophrenia that has not responded to other medications, but it requires frequent monitoring of white blood cells (Marder & Wirshing, 2009).

Difficulties with the side effects of clozapine led pharmaceutical companies to develop medications that might have the benefits of clozapine without its potentially fatal side effect of dramatic white blood count declines. A new series of SGAs was introduced with this hope. None of the SGA medications developed after clozapine caused severe white blood cell declines, but they all had remnants of the difficulties with side effects found in FGAs and none was as effective as clozapine in treating schizophrenia. Nonetheless, SGAs were regarded as an advance over FGAs because they had fewer EPS side effects and because they seemed to help schizophrenic patients' ability to interact with others. For the past several years the SGAs have been prescribed for children, adolescents, and adults at a much higher rate than have the FGAs (Olfson et al., 2006).

Risperidone serves as a good example to illustrate many of the strengths and weaknesses of SGA medications. Clinical trials of risperidone began in 1986, and the drug was approved by the FDA in 1994 as a treatment for adult patients with schizophrenia. Numerous studies have demonstrated that risperidone is effective in the treatment of adult schizophrenia (Goff, 2009). Compared to FGAs, risperidone and other SGAs are better accepted by patients, but they still have many side effects in common (Robinson et al., 2006).

As in the treatment of schizophrenia, risperidone works well in the treatment of adult bipolar disorder. Three large double-blind studies confirm that it is effective in adult bipolar disorder. Alone it works as well as lithium (Hirschfeld et al., 2004; Khanna et al., 2005). In other studies it has been shown to work well when given with lithium to adult bipolar disorder patients who did not respond to lithium alone (Sachs et al., 2002; Yatham et al., 2003). Like most currently marketed FGAs and SGAs, risperidone is FDA approved for the treatment of adult bipolar disorder. In children and adolescents it is FDA approved for use in schizophrenia in ages 13–17, the irritability associated with autism in ages 5 through 16, and for bipolar disorder in ages 10 through 17.

Although less frequent than occur with FGAs, risperidone does cause EPS side effects in adults, adolescents, and children. These side effects are related to the dose; the higher the dose of risperidone, the higher the rate of EPS side effects.

Another important side effect of risperidone and all antipsychotic medication is neuroleptic malignant syndrome, a rare but potentially deadly condition that requires immediate medical treatment. Neuroleptic malignant syndrome is characterized by muscle rigidity, fever, and changes in blood chemistry. It usually begins in the first two weeks of FGA or SGA treatment and is most common in the summer months. It can have up to a 30% death rate.

A less alarming side effect of many antipsychotic medications is weight gain; risperidone is associated with weight gain of about one-half pound per month. Over the long term, weight gain of this magnitude is a potentially serious health problem. Excessive weight gain from antipsychotic medications is associated with the development of a recently named side effect called the "metabolic syndrome," which includes the development of diabetes and increases in fats in the blood, including cholesterol. There are a variety of strategies for helping to prevent or minimize this weight gain.

Risperidone also has a variety of deleterious effects on sexual functioning. Fifteen percent of men experience sexual dysfunction or breast swelling on risperidone; 8% to 12% of women experience a loss of periods and/or the development of milk production and leakage. The side effects are caused by an increase in the hormone prolactin that is associated with pregnancy in normal female adults. Of interest, these sexual effects are not limited to adults: the prolactin increase associated with risperidone may be linked to breast size increase and (rarely) milk production in children of both sexes. Risperidone is associated with higher prolactin levels than occur with other SGAs. In addition to the sexual side effects, high prolactin levels have been associated with bone weakness. As with other medications in this chapter, at this time there are no research data regarding the long-term side effect of elevated levels of prolactin in children (Wieck & Haddad, 2004).

Some side effects of SGAs are more severe in children than in adults. Four SGAs, including risperidone, lead to more weight gain in children than in adults (Correll & Carlson, 2006; Safer, 2004). Children and adolescents are also more prone to Parkinsonian symptoms of EPS than adults (Correll & Schenk, 2008). The age of the patient is recognized as being a factor in the likelihood of tardive dyskinesia—youth is a relative protective factor and advanced age is a risk factor. In the elderly, the incidence of tardive dyskinesia is about 30% per year, whereas in young adults the incidence is about 5% (Correll & Schenk, 2008; Correll & Kane, 2007). Tardive dyskinesia seems to be less common in children than in adults. In a recent study of children who had taken SGAs for one year or less, 0.4% had developed tardive dyskinesia, which is lower than what has been reported for adults (Correll & Kane, 2007). The children were aged 4 to 18 and disproportionately male and white. There were 783 children studied in trials of SGAs, and three developed tardive dyskinesia. The symptoms of tardive dyskinesia disappeared in a matter of weeks in two of the children; there was no information about the third child. While this might initially seem encouraging, any reassurance gained by the relatively low rate of tardive dyskinesia and its apparent reversibility is offset by the brief time frame of the study. The risk of tardive dyskinesia continues to loom over the use of antipsychotics in children and adolescents.

Given the side effects of antipsychotics, it might be expected that mental health consumers and psychiatrists would minimize their use. Instead, their use has been increasing dramatically. From 1993 to 2002, according to a study conducted by Mark Olfson, MD, of Columbia University and his colleagues, the number of antipsychotics given to children and teenagers for mental health conditions increased by 600% (Olfson et al., 2006). In 1993 there were 201,000 child and adolescent outpatient visits at which antipsychotics were prescribed; in 2002 that number had risen to 1,224,000. Disruptive behavior disorders (ADHD, ODD conduct disorder) accounted for 37.8% of the prescriptions; mood disorder (bipolar disorder and depression) for 31.8%; developmental disorders (mental retardation and autism) for 17.3%; and psychotic disorders for 14.2%. Ninety-two percent of the antipsychotics were SGAs. Although these drugs have been recently approved for autism, bipolar disorder, and schizophrenia, their increase in use may also be related to a false sense of security about their freedom from side effects. Unfortunately, as described above, the SGAs do have a wide array of side effects. The apparent low rate in tardive dyskinesia in short-term studies does not mean the SGAs can be used with impunity. Short-term and long-term risks remain threats that counsel restraint in their use.

Clinically, antipsychotics have always been a mainstay of treatment of severe aggression, and this is true for children and adolescents as well as adults. It is particularly true within institutions. Aggression is a main reason for admission to child psychiatric hospital units, juvenile detention facilities, and other child treatment residential institutions. The child psychiatry field continues to weigh the risks and benefits in the use of these medications (Pappadopulos et al., 2003; Schur et al., 2003).

The dramatic increase in the use of this class of medication may in part be related to the increase in the use of the diagnosis of bipolar disorder in children and adolescents. This diagnosis may serve to legitimize the use of antipsychotics for everyone involved in an aggressive child's care. The medications are understood as not given simply to reduce the aggression but rather to treat an underlying illness. While this false belief may give temporary comfort to those involved, an incorrect diagnosis is not helpful. It is preferable to tell the parents and child the simple truth that the medicine is needed to control the child's aggression.

CONCLUSION

All three classes of medication discussed have significant side effects, and the consequences of taking them over a lifetime are not known. They should only be used in those clinical situations in which there is good reason to believe that they will be helpful.

REFERENCES

Bowden, C. (2009). Valproate. In A. F. Schatzberg & C. B. Nemeroff (Eds.), *Textbook of Psychopharmacology*. Arlington: American Psychiatric Publishing. Inc.

Bowden, C. L., & McElroy, S. L. (1995). History of the development of valproate for treatment of bipolar disorder. *J Clin Psychiatry, 56*, Suppl 3, 3–5.

Campbell, M., Adams, P. B., Small, A. M., Karantaris, V., Silva, R. R., Shell, J., Perry, R., & Overall, J. E. (1995). Lithium in hospitalized aggressive children with conduct disorder: a double-blind and placebo-controlled study. *J Am Acad Child Adolesc Psychiatry, 34*(4), 445–453.

Campbell, M., Small, A. M., Green, W. H., Jennings, S. J., Perry, R., Bennett, W. G., & Anderson, L. (1984). Behavioral efficacy of haloperidol and lithium carbonate. A comparison in hospitalized aggressive children with conduct disorder. *Arch Gen Psychiatry, 41*(7), 650–656.

Carlson, G. A., Rapport, M. D., Pataki, C. S., & Kelly, K. L. (1992). Lithium in hospitalized children at 4 and 8 weeks: Mood, behavior and cognitive effects. *J Child Psychol Psychiatry, 33* (2), 411–425.

Cooper, W. O., Federspiel, C. F., Griffin, M. R., & Hickson, G. B. (1997). New use of anticonvulsant medications among children enrolled in the Tennessee Medicaid Program. *Arch Pediatr Adolesc Med, 151*(12), 1242–1246.

Correll, C. U., & Carlson, H. E. (2006). Endocrine and metabolic adverse effects of psychotropic medications in children and adolescents. *J Am Acad Child Adolesc Psychiatry, 45*(7), 771–791.

Correll, C. U., & Kane, J. M. (2007). One-year incidence rates of tardive dyskinesia in children and adolescents treated with second-generation antipsychotics: A systematic review. *J Child Adolesc Psychopharmacol, 17*(5), 647–656.

Correll, C. U., & Schenk, E. M. (2008). Tardive dyskinesia and new antipsychotics. *Curr Opin Psychiatry, 2* (2), 151–156.

Donovan, S. J., Stewart, J. W., Nunes, E. V., Quitkin, F. M., Parides, M., Daniel, W., Susser, E., & Klein, D. F. (2000). Divalproex treatment for youth with explosive temper and mood lability: A double-blind, placebo-controlled crossover design. *Am J Psychiatry, 157*(5), 818–820.

Dursun, S., Haddad, P.M., & Barnes, T.R.E. (2004). Extrapyramidal Syndromes. In P. Haddad, S. Dursin, & B. Deakin (Eds.), *Adverse Syndromes and Psychiatric Drugs*. Oxford: Oxford University Press.

Findling, R. L., Frazier, J. A., Karantaris, V., Kowatch, R., McClellan, J., Pavuluri, M., Sikich, L., Hlastala, S., Hooper, S. R., Demeter, C. A., Bedoya, D., Brownstein, B., & Taylor-Zapata, P. (2008). The Collaborative Lithium Trials (CoLT): Specific aims, methods, and implementation. *Child Adolesc Psychiatry Ment Health, 2*(1), 21.

Findling, R. L., McNamara, N. K., Gracious, B. L., Youngstrom, E. A., Stansbrey, R. J., Reed, M. D., Demeter, C. A., Branicky, L. A., Fisher, K. E., & Calabrese, J. R. (2003). Combination lithium and divalproex sodium in pediatric bipolarity. *J Am Acad Child Adolesc Psychiatry, 42*(8), 895–901.

Findling, R. L., McNamara, N. K., Stansbrey, R., Gracious, B. L., Whipkey, R. E., Demeter, C. A., Reed, M. D., Youngstrom, E. A., & Calabrese, J. R. (2006). Combination lithium and divalproex sodium in pediatric bipolar symptom restabilization. *J Am Acad Child Adolesc Psychiatry, 45*(2), 142–148.

Findling, R. L., McNamara, N. K., Youngstrom, E. A., Stansbrey, R., Gracious, B. L., Reed, M. D., & Calabrese, J. R. (2005). Double-blind 18-month trial of lithium versus divalproex maintenance treatment in pediatric bipolar disorder. *J Am Acad Child Adolesc Psychiatry , 44*(5), 409–417.

Freeman, M. P., Wiegand, C.B., & Gelenberg, A. J. (2009). Lithium. In A. F. Schatzberg and C. B. Nemeroff (Eds.), *APA Textbook of Psychopharmacology*. Washington, DC: American Psychiatric Publishing, Inc.

Geller, B., Cooper, T. B., Sun, K., Zimerman, B., Frazier, J., Williams, M., et al. (1998). Double-blind and placebo-controlled study of lithium for adolescent bipolar disorders with secondary substance dependency. J Am Acad Child Adolesc Psychiatry, 37(2), 171–178.

Georgotas, A., & Gershon, S. (1981). Historical perspectives and current highlights on lithium treatment in manic-depressive illness. *J Clin Psychopharmacol, 1*(1), 27–31.

Goff, D. (2009). Risperidone and Paliperidone. In A. E. Schatzberg and C. B. Nemeroff (Eds.), *The American Psychiatric Publishing Textbook of Psychopharmacology*. Arlington: American Psychiatric Publishing, Inc.

Goodwin, F. K., & Jamison, K. R. (2007a). Medical Treatment of Depression. In F. K. Goodwin and J. K. Redfield (Eds.), *Manic-Depressive Illness: Bipolar Disorders and Recurrent Depression*. Oxford: Oxford University Press.

Goodwin, F. K., & Jamison, K. R. (2007b). Medical Treatment of Hypomania, Mania, and Mixed States. In F. K. Goodwin and J. K. Redfield (Eds.), *Manic-Depressive Illness: Bipolar Disorders and Recurrent Depression*. Oxford: Oxford University Press.

Hirschfeld, R. M., Keck, P. E., Jr., Kramer, M., Karcher, K., Canuso, C., Eerdekens, M., & Grossman, F. (2004). Rapid antimanic effect of risperidone monotherapy: A 3-week multicenter, double-blind, placebo-controlled trial. *Am J Psychiatry, 161*(6), 1057–1065.

Hunkeler, E. M., Fireman, B., & Lee, J. (2005). Trends in use of antidepressants, lithium and anticonvulsants in Kaiser Permante–insured youths, 1994–2003. *J Child Adolesc Psychopharmacol, 15*, 26–37.

Joffe, H., Cohen, L.S., Suppes, T., McLaughlin, W.L., Lavori, P., Adams, J.M., Hwang, C.H.,. Hall, J. E, & Sachs, G.S. (2006). Valproate is associated with new-onset oligoamenorrhea with hyperandrogenism in women with bipolar disorder. *Biol Psychiatry, 59*(11), 1078–1086.

Johnson, G., & Gershon, S. (1999). Early North American research on lithium. *Aust N Z J Psychiatry, 33 Suppl*, S48-53.

Kafantaris, V., Coletti, D.J., Dicker, R., Padula, G., Pleak, R.R., & Alvir, J.M. (2004). Lithium treatment of acute mania in adolescents: A placebo-controlled discontinuation study. *J Am Acad Child Adolesc Psychiatry, 43*(8), 984–993.

Khanna, S., Vieta, E., Lyons, B., Grossman, F., Eerdekens, M., & Kramer, M. (2005). Risperidone in the treatment of acute mania: Double-blind, placebo-controlled study. *Br J Psychiatry, 187*, 229–234.

Klein, R. G. (1991). Lithium effects in conduct disorders. In *CME Syllabus and Proceedings Summary, Symposium 2, 144th Annual Meeting of the American Psychiatric Assoc.* New Orleans, May11–16.

Kowatch, R.A., Suppes, T., Carmody, T.J., Bucci, J.P., Hume, J.H., Kromelis, M., Emslie, G.J., Weinberg , W.A., & Rush, A.J. (2000). Effect size of lithium, divalproex sodium, and carbamazepine in children and adolescents with bipolar disorder. *J Am Acad Child Adolesc Psychiatry, 39*(6), 713–720.

Malone, R.P., Delaney, M.A., Luebbert, J.F., Cater, J., & Campbell, M. (2000). A double-blind placebo-controlled study of lithium in hospitalized aggressive children and adolescents with conduct disorder. *Arch Gen Psychiatry, 57*(7), 649–654.

Marder, S. R., & Wirshing, D. A. (2009). Clozapine. In A.F. Schatzberg & C.B. Nemeroff (Eds.), *Textbook of Psychopharmacology*. Arlington: American Psychiatric Publishing, Inc.

Mitchell, P.B., & Hadzi-Pavlovic, D. (1999). John Cade and the discovery of lithium treatment for manic depressive illness. *Med J Aust, 171*(5), 262–264.

Nasrallah, H.A., & Tandon, R. (2009). Classic Antipsychotic Medication. In A.E. Schatzberg & C.B. Nemeroff (Eds.), *The American Psychiatric Publishing Textbook of Psychopharmacology*. Arlington: American Psychiatric Publishing, Inc.

Olfson, M., Blanco, C., Liu, L., Moreno, C., & Laje, G. (2006). National trends in the outpatient treatment of children and adolescents with antipsychotic drugs. *Arch Gen Psychiatry, 63*(6), 679–685.

Papatheodorou, G., Kutcher, S. P., Katic, M., & Szalai, J. P. (1995). The efficacy and safety of divalproex sodium in the treatment of acute mania in adolescents and young adults: An open clinical trial. *J Clin Psychopharmacol, 15*(2), 110–116.

Pappadopulos, E., MacIntyre, J. C. II, Crismon, M. L., Findling, R. L., Malone, R. P., Derivan, A., Schooler, N., Sikich, L., Greenhill, L., Schur, S. B., Felton, C. J., Kranzler, H., Rube, D. M., Sverd, J., Finnerty, M., Ketner, S., Siennick, S. E., & Jensen, P. S. (2003). Treatment recommendations for the use of antipsychotics for aggressive youth (TRAAY). Part II. *J Am Acad Child Adolesc Psychiatry, 42*(2), 145–161.

Pavuluri, M. N., Henry, D. B., Carbray, J. A., Sampson, G. A., Naylor, M. W., & Janicak, P. G. (2006). A one-year open-label trial of risperidone augmentation in lithium nonresponder youth with preschool-onset bipolar disorder. *J Child Adolesc Psychopharmacol, 16* (3), 336–350.

Pavuluri, M. N., Henry, D. B., Carbray, J. A., Sampson, G. A., Naylor, M. W., & Janicak, P. G. (2004). Open-label prospective trial of risperidone in combination with lithium or divalproex sodium in pediatric mania. *J Affect Disord, 82*, Suppl 1, S103–111.

Rifkin, A., Karajgi, B., Dicker, R., Perl, E., Boppana, V., Hasan, N., & Pollack, S. (1997). Lithium treatment of conduct disorders in adolescents. *Am J Psychiatry, 154*(4), 554–555.

Robinson, D. G., Woerner, M. G., Napolitano, B., Patel, R. C., Sevy, S. M., Gunduz-Bruce, H., Soto-Perello, J. M., Mendelowitz, A., Khadivi, A., Miller, R., McCormack, J., Lorell, B. S., Lesser, M. L., Schooler, N. R., & Kane, J. M. (2006). Randomized comparison of olanzapine versus risperidone for the treatment of first-episode schizophrenia: 4-month outcomes. *Am J Psychiatry, 16* (12), 2096–2102.

Rosenthal, N. E., & Goodwin, F. K. (1982). The role of the lithium ion in medicine. *Annu Rev Med, 33*, 555–568.

Sachs, G. S., Grossman, F., Ghaemi, S. N., Okamoto, A., & Bowden, C. L. (2002). Combination of a mood stabilizer with risperidone or haloperidol for treatment of acute mania: A double-blind, placebo-controlled comparison of efficacy and safety. *Am J Psychiatry, 159*(7), 1146–1154.

Safer, D. J. (2004). A comparison of risperidone-induced weight gain across the age span. *J Clin Psychopharmacol, 24*(4), 429–436.

Schur, S. B., Sikich, L., Findling, R. L., Malone, R. P., Crismon, M. L., Derivan, A., MacIntyre, J. C. II, Pappadopulos, E., Greenhill, L., Schooler, N., Van Orden, K., & Jensen, P. S. (2003). Treatment recommendations for the use of antipsychotics for aggressive youth (TRAAY). Part I: A review. *J Am Acad Child Adolesc Psychiatry, 42*(2), 132–144.

Steiner, H., K. Saxena, & Chang, K. (2003). Psychopharmacologic strategies for the treatment of aggression in juveniles. *CNS Spectr, 8*(4), 298–308.

Wagner, K. D., Kowatch, R. A., Emslie, G. J., Findling, R. L., Wilens, T. E., McCague, K., D'Souza, J., Wamil, A., Lehman, R. B., Berv, D., & Linden, D. (2006). A double-blind, randomized, placebo-controlled trial of oxcarbazepine in the treatment of bipolar disorder in children and adolescents. *Am J Psychiatry, 163*(7), 1179–1186.

West, S. A., Keck, P. E. Jr., & McElroy, S. L. (1994). Open trial of valproate in the treatment of adolescent mania. *J. Child Adolesc Psychopharmacol, 4*, 263–267.

Wieck, A., & Haddad, P.M. (2004). Hyperprolactinaemia. In P. Haddad, S. Dursin, & B. Deakin (Eds.), *Adverse Syndromes and Psychiatric Drugs*. Oxford: Oxford University Press.

Yatham, L. N., Grossman, F., Augustyns, I., Vieta, E., & Ravindran, A. (2003). Mood stabilisers plus risperidone or placebo in the treatment of acute mania. International, double-blind, randomised controlled trial. *Br J Psychiatry, 182*, 141–147.

Zito, J. M., Safer, D. J., Gardner, J. F., Soeken, K., & Ryu, J. (2006). Anticonvulsant treatment for psychiatric and seizure indications among youths. *Psychiatr Serv, 57*(5), 681–685.

8

Clinical Trials

Misdeeds of the pharmaceutical industry have been denounced recently in books, the press, and Congress (Angell, 2004). At the highest organizational levels, some drug companies have engaged in unethical conduct. These practices have included minimizing or concealing dangerous side effects, exaggerating treatment benefits, and exerting undue influence on psychiatric and other mental health professionals. Drug companies have also engaged in a number of other breaches of trust, as documented in many books and articles written about the subject. Marcia Angell, MD, former editor of the *New England Journal of Medicine* and a well-known critic of the pharmaceutical industry, concluded her review of three books criticizing American psychiatry and the pharmaceutical industry by stating, "It is simply no longer possible to believe much of the clinical research that is published, or to rely on the judgment of trusted physicians or authoritative medical guidelines. I take no pleasure in this conclusion" (Angell, 2009, p. 12).

I do not wish to contest the fact that unethical conduct has occurred, as it has in other corporations and institutions in America, such the banking industry, the oil industry, and the tobacco industry, to mention just a few. It is also the case that within the pharmaceutical industry there are a large number of dedicated and ethical scientists who pursue efforts to assess the effects of medications on mental illness with the best techniques available. The political and public outrage surrounding the behaviors of the unethical few has had an impact on the credibility of the industry as a whole. Unfortunately, it has jeopardized the industry's ability to gain public support for the medication treatment of child psychiatric illness.

I want to express a limited dissent to the constant vilification of pharmaceutical companies. My dissent will be in part based on a personal reminiscence of the progress in clinical child psychiatry since I began as a trainee in the field in 1967 and will also include a brief consideration of the conduct of clinical trials. In the concluding portion of this chapter, I will discuss a clinical trial of one of the medications commonly prescribed for pediatric bipolar disorder.

A CHANGE IN CLINICAL CHILD PSYCHIATRY

In 1967, the primary form of treatment for child psychiatric disorders was psychoanalysis or psychoanalytically oriented play therapy. This consisted largely of interpreting children's play in individual play therapy sessions. The therapy was nonspecific; that is, each child was treated largely the same way based on psychoanalytic concepts regardless of the child's difficulty. The children were often seen several times per week. Some children seemed to improve over time, but a large number did not.

During this time, angry, disruptive children were frequently placed outside of the home for long stays in hospitals or other residential facilities. Part of my own training included supervised treatment of psychiatrically hospitalized children seen four times per week in individual play therapy. The children were in residence in this highly regarded psychiatric training institution for one to several years.

For the parents and children, the treatment was lengthy (often measured in years), expensive, and only marginally effective. For the provider of the therapy, it was sometimes interesting but more often tedious and frustrating. Failure of the patient to improve after a lengthy period of time and the subsequent disappointment, sense of failure, anger, and recriminations from parents were substantial risks to this form of treatment for practitioners. After several years of practicing this type of therapy, many child psychiatrists of that era (1950–1980) left the field of child psychiatry for other branches of psychiatry

Of course, at times the treatment outcomes were rewarding. I once treated a seven-year-old boy named Jimmy, a verbal child who had come to treatment in the mid-1970s because of anxiety about attending school, fear of the dark, and concern about his ability to succeed in his academically demanding private elementary school. I saw him once a week for psychoanalytically oriented play therapy in a private office in my suburban home. Over a period of several months, we played innumerable games of checkers in which he managed to overcome his fear of competition and become more assertive. After drawing pictures and telling me stories based on his imaginings, he became more comfortable with his angry feelings and fears. He seemed to improve considerably over the several months of treatment, a relatively brief period of time for psychotherapy in that era. Toward the end of his therapy, he asked, "You know, Dr. Kaplan, I like coming here. We play together, we draw pictures, I tell you stories, but can you tell me, what do you do for a living?"

Though his question was, in part, an expression of a lack of intellectual understanding of the treatment, for many children not so fortunate as Jimmy the question might express a darker truth: this form of therapy lasted for years with little tangible benefit. The field of child mental health desperately needed specific, effective, and rapid treatments for child psychiatric problems.

After the *DSM-III* system was introduced in 1980, the use of appropriate medications, based on specific *DSM* criteria, dramatically increased the ability of child psychiatrists to be helpful to the children brought to them. Currently, in part as a result of the efforts of the pharmaceutical industry, we do have effective treatments. The majority of the patients I see are dramatically improved after only a handful of sessions. Contemporary approaches to treatment have reduced the length of stay in psychiatric hospitals for children from years to weeks to days. There are a variety of reasons for this apparent improvement in treatment outcomes, but my impression is that improved diagnostic criteria (the *DSM* system), medications targeted to those criteria, and drug-company-funded studies of the medications are largely responsible for the briefer and more effective treatments we see today.

The *DSM-III* and more recent *DSM-IV* systems have provided psychiatrists with a basis for diagnosis and a rationale for effective use of medicines developed by the pharmaceutical industry. A child with a particular *DSM* diagnosis is more likely to respond to a medication meant for that diagnosis than a medication not meant for that diagnosis. For example, a child diagnosed with ADHD using *DSM* criteria should be given a medicine that has been shown to be effective for that disorder, such as stimulant medications (methylphenidate, amphetamines, etc.), rather than a medication shown to be effective for another disorder; a child diagnosed with a *DSM* anxiety disorder should be given a medication shown to be effective for that disorder, such as fluvoxamine (brand name Luvox) for obsessive-compulsive disorder. The doctor is driven to search for the correct diagnosis based on *DSM-IV* criteria to enable the correct medication to be prescribed.

Along with *DSM* diagnoses and contemporary psychopharmacology, psychotherapy has improved greatly as well. Cognitive therapy, family therapy, and behavior therapy have all increased the range and improved the effectiveness of interventions available for children. The use of medications is sometimes accompanied by a psychotherapeutic treatment effort and is sometimes accompanied by an educational intervention as well.

Arguably, it is often the medication that seems crucial in facilitating the improvement. These medications would not have been available except for the efforts of the pharmaceutical industry. Of course, the pharmaceutical industry had its own economic incentives for developing and studying these drugs. This separate agenda does not diminish the experience of the mental health consumer, who benefits greatly from the medications for mental illness developed through pharmaceutical company efforts.

This is not meant to gloss over the difficulties of the many children who do not respond to currently available treatment efforts or who only partially respond. The violent, depressed, anxious, or psychotic children who fail to respond to treatment suffer greatly and break the hearts of their families and the professionals who labor to help them. The need for better medications, better psychotherapy approaches, and better approaches to diagnosis is painfully obvious to those of us who work with these children and their families.

INTRODUCTION TO CLINICAL TRIALS

The clinical trial is at the core of the science of clinical psychiatry and is intimately related to the clinical scientific enterprise of the pharmaceutical industry. It is a frequently mentioned and often criticized topic in the popular press, yet my impression is that there is little public understanding about what actually takes place during such a trial. It should be useful, therefore, to provide some introductory information about both the goals and the processes of the clinical trial.

The purpose of a clinical trial is to study whether a medication reduces the symptoms of an illness safely. In psychiatry trials and most medical trials, patients receive either the drug being tested or a lookalike pill called a placebo. Clinical trials need placebos because many people feel better just because they have taken a pill, even if it is simply a sugar pill. This is called the "placebo effect," and it is a critical issue in the study of psychiatric medication because the treatment effect of the medication is often small and the placebo effect is often large. In clinical trials, for the medication to be considered to work, it must help more than the placebo. Clinical trials help to ensure that any changes in the illness are due to the medication and not to the placebo effect.

To clarify this, let's examine more closely the actual mechanics of one such study, the double-blind, parallel-group, randomized trial, which is the gold standard of psychiatric clinical trials. In this design neither the patient nor the doctor knows whether the patient is receiving the medication or the placebo. The patient and doctor are both "blind" to what the patient is taking—hence the term "double-blind." "Parallel groups" refers to the fact that the patients who receive the placebo are treated exactly the same as the patients who receive the medication. The study runs parallel for the two groups, and members of each receive the same procedures, have the same number of visits, and are asked the same questions; everything about the experience of the patients is identical except for the medication. One critical aspect of this type of trial is that the patients must be put into the placebo or medication groups by chance. This critical process, called "randomization," ensures that the patients are the same at the beginning of the study and that there is a minimum of difference between the two groups on measures of social class, race, IQ, illness severity, and an infinite number of other attributes that may influence the response to the medication or placebo. The importance of the randomization process to the scientific value of clinical trials cannot be overemphasized.

In an "open," nonblind clinical trial, on the other hand, both the doctor and the patient know that the patient is receiving medication, and no placebos are used. Though these studies can be useful, they are not considered as thorough or credible as the double-blind, placebo-controlled, parallel-group, randomized trial described above. Most significantly, when the study doctors know that the patients are taking a medication they run the risk of being predisposed to rate the patients as showing improvement. It is not necessary to imagine any dishonesty on the part of the doctors; their beliefs and enthusiasm about the medication may unconsciously lead them to report improvement. Similarly, the patients, knowing that they are receiving medication for their illness, may also be predisposed to view themselves as improved. This is a natural phenomenon in clinical trials and is the reason placebos are so important.

MULTISITE CLINICAL TRIALS

For technical reasons that needn't be discussed here, clinical trials often require a large number of patients—more than could be obtained by one doctor alone. For this reason, most clinical trials use many doctors at many sites or locations simultaneously. The trials at these different sites must be closely coordinated. In studies with doctors at many locations, called "multisite studies," a considerable amount of activity takes place before the first patient is admitted to the study and randomized.

First, a meeting is held for all of the doctors and clinical staff from each of the sites that will be performing the trial. The purpose of the meeting is to ensure that the doctors and clinical staff understand how the study is to be conducted. Lectures are provided about the administrative arrangements of the trial and the medication to be used. Often, a central focus of the meeting is the symptom rating scales. The goal is to ensure that the doctors and clinical staff use the scales the same way and score patients the same way at each site. Usually, lectures are given about the rating instruments, films are shown of patients with the disorder to be studied, and the instrument ratings of the patient shown in the film are discussed. Finally, a videotape of a patient is shown as a test, and the doctors and other clinical staff must be similar in how they rate the patient with the instrument. If a doctor or clinical staff rater is not able to rate the patient correctly, he or she may not be allowed to participate in the trial or may be allowed to try to rate again on a different tape. Ensuring that all the study-site personnel behave similarly allows for information from the different sites to be combined.

After this initial meeting, doctors and clinical staff at the sites use the research instruments to examine patients to ensure that the patients have the diagnosis with which the study is concerned. If the purpose of the double-blind trial is to examine the ability of a medication to be helpful with bipolar disorder, for example, it is essential that the patients have bipolar disorder and that all of the doctors at all of the sites have decided this in the same way.

Patients who meet the diagnostic and other criteria may then move on to be assigned to placebo or medication by chance; that is, "randomized." In clinical trials, the patients usually are randomized by a central location rather than by the doctor seeing the patient. The doctor and staff are given a code that matches a code on the blinded study drug and do not know whether the code indicates the medication or the placebo. The pills look the same. This keeps the staff and doctor blind to who is receiving the drug and who is receiving the placebo, and it ensures that the patients are assigned by chance to either group.

Examination of the patients during the patients' trial visits is comprehensive. Generally, numerous interviews are given at each visit. Questionnaires are given to children, parents, and sometimes teachers as well. Side effects are evaluated, and no effort is spared to provide the highest-quality care to the children receiving either the drug or the placebo. Ethics committees oversee all aspects of the trials. Trial personnel expend great effort in rating the symptoms over the course of the trial to obtain the most accurate data possible. It is surprising how difficult it can be even for very experienced clinicians to distinguish between who is getting the medication and who is getting the placebo. The study clinicians are encouraged to focus on rating the symptoms of the patient's behavior on the questionnaires rather than attempting to guess who is getting the placebo and who is getting the medication.

Typically, studies are also monitored by outside agencies such as ethics committees, pharmaceutical companies, or other companies hired to ensure the integrity of the study. For many studies, the Food and Drug Administration (FDA) oversees the conduct of the trial. Study sites are examined for various administrative mandates, such as proper laboratory facilities and properly qualified clinical staff. Many times, the clinicians' adherence to the proper use of the research interview assessments, as taught in the initial meeting, is scrutinized over the length of the trial. The physical presence of outside auditors and monitors reviewing records and interviewing personnel is a frequent occurrence at clinical trial sites.

Often, at the end of the study, the performance of sites is compared to learn which sites performed best. Careful symptom rating enables sites to have data that are more likely to separate placebo from medication if the medication works. Sites that performed well are likely to be invited to participate in future trials.

Compare the usual clinical psychiatric care provided in an outpatient setting with the care provided during a clinical trial. In the outpatient setting the typical initial evaluation lasts about an hour and physical assessment of the patients' medical status is minimal; in the clinical trial, the initial assessment can last several hours and includes an exhaustive physical assessment of the patient's medical status. In addition, standardized rating instruments and assessment scales are used at every session in the clinical trial, though they are rarely used at all in the outpatient clinical setting. In clinical settings, beyond monetary constraints imposed by insurance companies, there is minimal outside auditing to ensure that adequate treatment is taking place. Clinicians are largely free to do as they please. In contrast, the clinical trial setting is highly structured and monitored.

To evaluate clinical trials on pediatric bipolar disorder it is important to understand some of the concepts on which the studies are based.

EXAMPLE OF A CLINICAL TRIAL

An influential study of valproate (brand name Depakote) in children diagnosed with bipolar disorder will serve to illustrate many of the principles of the double-blind clinical trial.

In 2006 an industry-funded double-blind, placebo-controlled clinical trial of valproate was conducted for pediatric bipolar disorder (Wagner et al., 2009). There was reason to believe that this medication might work in pediatric bipolar disorder: it had worked in some open studies, it worked in placebo-controlled double-blind studies for adults, and it had worked in one double-blind controlled trial for children and adolescents with bipolar disorder (Kowatch et al., 2000). The 2006 study will be reviewed in detail because of its unexpected outcome and its potential importance in the development of professional reservations about the status of pediatric bipolar disorder.

In every double-blind clinical trial, the "primary efficacy measure" is the one measure that must improve to conclude that the medication worked. This measure must be selected before the trial begins. Many other measures made during the trial may have worked or failed to work, but the success of the tested agent to treat a disorder depends on how well the agent works on the primary outcome measure. For pediatric bipolar disorder clinical trials the primary outcome measure is invariably the Young Mania Rating Scale or YMRS (pronounced "why-mars") (Young et al., 1978). This scale is used in most adult studies of bipolar disorder as well. It is an easy symptom checklist to complete and provides a measure of the presence and severity of bipolar disorder. As shown in Table 8.1, the YMRS has 11 symptoms. As shown in Table 8.2, each of these symptoms is assessed according to the degree to which it is present in the patient. For example, in the case of symptom #1, Elevated Mood, a patient may exhibit anything from total absence of elevated mood (0) to euphoria, inappropriate laughter, and/or singing (4).

All clinical trials list specific inclusion criteria to describe exactly who will be allowed into the study. Among the inclusion criteria for this study were children and adolescents between the ages of 10 and 17 with a diagnosis of bipolar disorder or mixed episode and a YMRS score of 20 or more. "Mixed episode," according to the *DSM-IV*, means that the "criteria are met for both a manic episode and for a major depressive episode nearly every day during at least a 1-week period" (American Psychiatric Association, 2000, p. 365).

The diagnosis was made with the K-SADS. As in any medication study, there were also conditions that excluded patients from participating. The long list of exclusions for this study included, among other things, drug abuse, intellectual disability, and current violent or current suicidal behavior. Patients who had ADHD were permitted to take stimulants, but other medications directly related to the treatment of bipolar disorder were excluded.

The double-blind trial lasted for four weeks and was followed by a six-month open trial in which everyone who completed the double-blind

TABLE 8.1. Young Mania Rating Scale (YMRS) Items

1. Elevated Mood
2. Increased Motor Activity
3. Sexual Interest
4. Sleep
5. Irritability
6. Speech
7. Language/Thought Disorder
8. Content
9. Disruptive/Aggressive
10. Appearance
11. Insight

(From Young, R. C., Biggs, J. T., Ziegler, V. E., & Meyer, D. A. [1978]. A rating scale for mania. *British Journal of Psychiatry*, 133, 429–435. (c) 1978 The Royal College of Psychiatrics. Reprinted with permission.)

TABLE 8.2. Example of the 1–4 Scoring Choices for a YMRS Item (YMRS Item #1)

1. Elevated Mood
   0 Absent
   1 Mildly or possibly increased on questioning
   2 Definite subjective elevation; optimistic, self-confident; cheerful; appropriate to content
   3 Elevated; inappropriate to content; humorous
   4 Euphoric; inappropriate laughter; singing

trial had the opportunity to receive the medication. An open trial of this sort affords investigators the opportunity to learn more about the longer-term side effects of a medication and to learn more about how well the drug works over a longer period of time.

One hundred and fifty-one patients began the study; 77 patients were assigned by randomization to the valproate group and 74 were assigned to the placebo group. Fifty-six patients completed the study in the valproate group and 61 completed the study in the placebo group. Sixty-six patients (31 from the valproate group and 35 from the placebo group) enrolled in the six-month, long-term, open-study portion, and 26 patients completed it.

At the beginning of the study, weekly during the double-blind portion, and monthly during the long-term open study, the patients were rated on the YMRS. Ratings were based on behavior for the previous seven days. At the beginning of the study, before the medication was taken, the average YMRS score was 31.3 for the placebo group and 31.0 for the valproate group. A 50% decrease in the YMRS was defined as indicating that the drug had worked.

Over the four-week double-blind study the YMRS of the placebo group declined (improved) 7.9 points, and the valproate group declined (improved) 8.8 points. There was no meaningful difference between the two improvement scores either statistically or clinically. In other words, the patients who got the placebo improved as much as the patients who got the valproate. Only 24% of the valproate group were responders (showed a 50% reduction in YMRS score), and 23% of the placebo group were responders. Again, there was no meaningful difference between the placebo group and the valproate group in the percent of responders.

The valproate didn't work. This finding was unexpected. Valproate had been widely used for the clinical treatment of pediatric bipolar disorder. Its failure to work in a large, carefully done, placebo-controlled, double-blind trial may have been an unpleasant surprise to the many psychiatrists, child psychiatrists, and pediatricians who prescribed it to children regularly. Prescribing any medication involves a careful weighing of risks and benefits; as was described in chapter 7, valproate has a lot of potential side effects. After the results of the valproate study were published, it became difficult to justify the use of a medication that had little scientific evidence to support its benefits and much scientific evidence to support its risks.

The failure of valproate to separate from placebo in the trial may have dealt an important psychological blow to the acceptance of the disorder for the practicing clinician. As a measure of distress in the professional child psychiatric community about the failure of valproate to work in this trial, Dr. Robert Kowatch, a distinguished researcher in the pharmacologic treatment of pediatric bipolar disorder, warned in a widely circulated book chapter:

This trial may have may have had negative results because the active treatment period of four weeks was not long enough or because the serum [blood] levels of valproate were not high enough. The result of one possibly negative study of valproate in children and adolescents with bipolar disorder must be interpreted with caution and child psychiatrists should not stop using valproate until there is more in-depth examination of this trial and subsequent replications. (Kowatch, 2009, p. 140)

Published complaints about the techniques of performing or interpreting the result of a trial rarely surface in print in the American psychiatric community. This complaint was especially unusual in that Dr. Kowatch was an author of the study.

Despite Dr. Kowatch's complaint, the blood levels of valproate were carefully reported in the study and were adequate. As to the timing being too short, Dr. Kowatch neglects to mention that the six-month open portion of the study also did not improve the symptoms of bipolar disorder; the YMRS only dropped little more than two points during this extra time on the drug. Six months is a more-than-adequate length of time to study the effect of a medication. Dr. Kowatch's characterization of this double-blind, placebo-controlled study as "one possibly negative study" unfairly minimizes the singular importance of this study. As has been discussed extensively, double-blind, placebo-controlled studies are the gold standard of clinical effectiveness. They take precedence over open studies and have much greater scientific weight.

Having addressed the failure of valproate to improve the symptoms of pediatric bipolar disorder any more than did a placebo, consider the side effects of valproate during this trial. The FDA demands efficacy (proof that the drug works compared to a placebo) and safety before granting approval of the drug to be marketed for a specific patient group; in this case, children. The safety of a medication receives intense scrutiny during the conduct of a clinical trial. A considerable amount of bureaucracy and bureaucratic jargon have developed in association with concerns about medication side effects and the FDA approval process. Because no one can be sure whether a physical symptom is due to the medication under study, patients in clinical trials are watched for any kind of medical event, and the events are compared for the patients on the medication and the patients on the placebo. In the valproate trial, there were several medical problems that occurred more in the children who received valproate than in the children who received a placebo.

There were differences in weight gain over the four-week double-blind study. The valproate group gained 4.4 pounds, and the placebo group gained 0.66 pounds. The difference was significant statistically and clinically. There are considerable risks of gaining about one pound per week, including diabetes, heart disease, hypertension, and other disorders associated with obesity. There were also differences in laboratory values from blood tests over the four-week study. The valproate group had a significant decrease in platelet count (the part of the blood responsible for clotting) compared to the placebo group and a significant increase in ammonia. Ammonia is a chemical found in normal blood, and it is well known that valproate raises its level. One child in the study had to be hospitalized because of a high ammonia level, and four children were noted to have toxic levels of ammonia.

As noted above, after the four-week double-blind study ended, all patients, from both the placebo group and the valproate group, were offered the opportunity to participate in a six-month study in which everyone received the valproate. Sixty-six patients enrolled in the long-term open study. Forty patients, or 61%, left the open phase of the study prematurely for a variety of reasons. Two children withdrew from the study because of baldness or hair loss, one for obesity, one for low platelet count, and one for increased ammonia. In general, the drug does not seem to have been well accepted by the parents and children.

These side effects are serious. As valproate did not improve manic symptoms in this pediatric bipolar disorder study, the risk of these serious side effects cannot be justified.

The failure of the valproate trial to work for pediatric bipolar disorder goes a small distance toward calling into question the diagnosis itself. If valproate works on bipolar disorder in adults yet does not work in children, some may question whether the children are truly suffering from the same disease.

CONCLUSION

Clinical trials that use double-blind, placebo-controlled, randomized methodology in children are necessary to demonstrate that medications work and are safe.

A carefully done industry-sponsored clinical trial can generate important information that can run counter to the financial interests of the sponsoring drug company and the expectations of the investigators in the trial.

REFERENCES

American Psychiatric Association. (2000). *Diagnostic and Statistical Manual of Mental Disorders.* 4th ed. Text Revision ed. Washington, DC: American Psychiatric Association.

Angell, M. (2004). *The Truth About the Drug Companies: How They Deceive Us and What to Do About It.* New York: Random House.

Angell, M. (2009, January 15). Drug Companies & Doctors: A Story of Corruption. *New York Review Of Books.*

Kowatch, R. A., Fristad, M.A., Findling, R.L., Post, R.M. (Ed.). (2009). *Clinical Manual for Management of Bipolar Disorder in Children and Adolescents.* Arlington, VA: American Psychiatric Publishing, Inc.

Kowatch, R.A., Suppes, T., Carmody, T.J., Bucci, J. P, Hume, J.H., Kromelis, M., Emslie, G.J., Weinberg, W.A., & Rush, A.J. (2000). Effect size of lithium, divalproex sodium, and carbamazepine in children and adolescents with bipolar disorder. *J Am Acad Child Adolesc Psychiatry* , *39* (6), 713–720.

Wagner, K.D., Redden, L., Kowatch, R.A., Wilens, T.E., Segal, S., Chang, K., Wozniak, P., Vigna, N.V., Abi-Saab, W., & Saltarelli, M. (2009). A double-blind, randomized, placebo-controlled trial of divalproex extended-release in the treatment of bipolar disorder in children and adolescents. *J Am Acad Child Adolesc Psychiatry, 48*(5), 519–532.

Young, R.C., Biggs, J.T., Ziegler, V.E., & Meyer, D.A. (1978). A rating scale for mania: Reliability, validity and sensitivity. *Br J Psychiatry, 133,* 429–435.

9

Bad Science

Most researchers who study pediatric bipolar disorder are passionate about their work. They believe in the existence of the disorder and in the great importance of describing, understanding, treating, and preventing it. Equipped with well-designed questionnaires, carefully selected patients, expert statistical analysis, and ample funding, exceptionally competent, scrupulously honest researchers have invested years in the study of a disorder that almost certainly does not exist.

The strength of the researchers' wish to find pediatric bipolar disorder seems to have led them to find it when it wasn't there. The situation may be analogous to the well-known Rorschach test in which patients are shown an ambiguous inkblot and are asked to describe what they see. Their perceptions are based in part on the actual form of the inkblot but are also strongly related to their inner beliefs and experiences. The welter of aggressive behaviors along with the many additional diagnoses these children have may have created an ambiguous situation for clinicians and investigators that made it more likely they would see what they wished to see.

Another analogy is a frequently told story from psychoanalytic training. Most psychoanalytic training is based largely on the theories of Sigmund Freud, who amongst many other things, developed the Oedipal theory of human development, which was based on the belief that all males had a wish to kill their fathers and marry their mothers. This wish is purportedly unconscious but can be brought to light during a Freudian psychoanalysis. Psychoanalytic trainees who could not find evidence for this in their patients, the story goes, were admonished by their instructors to keep looking; if they looked hard enough, they would find it. One interpretation of this anecdote is that the student analyst would find evidence of the Oedipal theory even if it were not there.

Contemporary investigators are not immune from seeing what they want to see. Although there are numerous research strategies to prevent this, these safeguards have not been enough to limit the wishes or perceptual distortions of many investigators of pediatric bipolar disorder.

This concern is not just an abstract issue for me. I have several times been requested to serve as an investigator in medication studies of pediatric bipolar disorder but declined because I knew that my colleagues would often see bipolar disorder in the research subjects and I would rarely if ever diagnose the disorder in potential research subjects. Simple perceptual bias in the observation of patients plays an important role in the high rates of pediatric bipolar disorder diagnoses.

THE IMPORTANCE OF FALSIFICATION

Hugh Heclo, Robinson Professor of Public Affairs at George Mason University School of Public Policy and member of the American Academy of Arts and Sciences, writes:

The scientific method requires human beings—the scientists who make up this community—who are positively committed to seeking contrary evidence and who reject any effort to protect scientific statements from falsification (for example, by changing definitions, bringing in ad hoc hypotheses, using authority to dismiss evidence, personally attacking critics, or suppressing inconvenient facts). . . . To reject this moral obligation to seek the truth through falsification is to abandon science itself and launch in to a different game. (Heclo 2008, p. 87)

The scientific spirit demands an active effort to falsify a hypothesis or theory and to take a skeptical attitude toward one's own findings. The scientist attempts to develop tests of the theory or hypothesis to disprove it. Initially, Einstein's theories about light and mass were greeted with skepticism because they were not believed to be falsifiable with the technology available at the time. Since they could not be disproven at the time they were announced, they were considered by some to not be scientific. Psychoanalytic theory has been regarded as unscientific because it can never be falsified or proven wrong.

In a similar vein, I recall a consultation I performed for a preschool program many years ago. The director of the program, a psychoanalyst, was a warm and wise person who knew each patient in the program very well. She wanted me to help develop a research program for the unit. As we toured the unit each week, the director frequently commented on the behaviors of various children in the program. No matter what the children were doing she would exclaim, "See? That proves that Freud was right." It was clear that to her there was no behavior that might possibly prove that Freud was wrong. In that setting, every behavior was reduced to a confirmation of Freud's beliefs. Scientific skepticism had no role in that unit and has had little role in the study of pediatric bipolar disorder.

Is there a study or experiment that might disprove the high rates of bipolar disorder in childhood reported over the past decade? Simple observation that the children don't look like adults with bipolar disorder has not been persuasive to the advocates of the childhood diagnosis. Neither has failure to find bipolar disorder in the children of adult bipolar disorder patients. Treatment studies provide little evidence to support the disorder in childhood, but this has not dissuaded the advocates, nor has failure to identify the disorder in epidemiologic studies of childhood.

Heclo observed that one method of avoiding falsification was by changing definitions. The advocates of pediatric bipolar disorder use changes in the definition of the disorder to advance their belief that the disorder exists and is more common than expected. The large number of redefinitions of bipolar disorder has been reviewed. By changing the definition of the disorder, advocates of the disorder in childhood report high rates of the diagnosis; none report its absence or rarity. As has been discussed, the redefinitions of bipolar disorder of the Biederman group (severe aggression) and the Geller group (grandiosity and elation) led to high rates of the disorder in their own groups' studies. The Geller redefinition of mood swings—calling them radian or ultraradian—was an obvious intrusion on the traditional vocabulary of the bipolar disorder diagnosis and allowed mood swings occurring 360 times per year to count as bipolar disorder cycles. Not to be ignored is the frequent use and redefinition of the bipolar disorder NOS category. The frequent redefinition of the bipolar diagnosis was an effort by the advocates to characterize bipolar disorder in childhood, but the multiple definitions inflated the rate of diagnosis of pediatric bipolar disorder (Ghaemi & Martin, 2007).

DIAGNOSTIC ERRORS

There are many sources of error in making a diagnosis. One source of error is redefining or failing to consistently apply *DSM* diagnostic criteria. A second source of error in making a diagnosis is the interview or questionnaire used to gather the information to make the diagnosis. Traditional clinical diagnostic psychiatric interviews vary a great deal by the theoretical orientation of the interviewer and the administrative requirements of the clinic.

For research, it is critically important that questions be asked and information gathered in a consistent fashion. To make information gathering more systematic, standardized research interviews were developed.

Standardized research interviews were a revolutionary advance in psychiatric mental health research technology in that they ensured the consistency of interviews from interviewer to interviewer and hospital to hospital. They specified each question the patient was asked and provided a code for each reply. The replies were tallied using interview rules, which then led to a *DSM* diagnosis. Structured psychiatric interviews are interviews in which every question has to be asked in the exact form in which it was written and replies have to be precisely coded in accord with the specific rules of the interview.

Semistructured interviews, in contrast, allow the written questions for each symptom to serve as only a suggestion for the interviewer. The interviewer is allowed to modify the question to make it more understandable to the patient. Also, the interviewer can develop his or her own follow-up questions, as needed, depending on what the patient said and whether the interviewer believed more information was needed. Suggestions are given for coding answers as well. The semistructured interview provided more freedom for the interviewer to pursue openings or leads provided by the patient. While most structured psychiatric interviews could be performed by nonprofessional or lay interviewers, semistructured interviews required an advanced degreed mental health professional because of the greater amount of judgment and experience required to perform the interview well.

An informative study that used a structured psychiatric interview— the Diagnostic Interview for Children, or DISC—is directly related to the measurement of pediatric bipolar disorder symptoms (Breslau, 1987). The DISC is designed to be given by nonprofessional interviewers. It was initially developed to assess the frequency of child mental health disorders in the community. The study looked at whether the interview was accurately coming up with diagnoses. The point of the study was to see if the DISC caused "false positives" (saying a person has a symptom when the person truly does not) or "false negatives" (saying a person does not have a symptom when the person truly does). For this study, each time the subjects gave a response, the interviewer asked the subject to give several examples, which were recorded. The interviewers did not use the examples to code the responses but coded the responses as they routinely did by following the interview rules. Later, the responses were reviewed by expert reviewers who compared the lay interview coding with the examples provided by the subjects. The lay interviewers following the rules of the DISC interview found that 11.5% of the child subjects were considered grandiose. After the experts reviewed the examples, the experts believed that only 0.4% of the child subjects were grandiose.

The two questions that were asked about grandiosity were, "Have you had some kind of special powers which make it possible for you to do things that other people your own age can't do?" and "Have you ever felt that you are one of the most important persons in the world?" Examples of positive replies falsely coded as grandiose on the interview are "I do the best work in my class; I read better than others" and "No one is more important to myself than me."

The authors note that thoughts that are often part of normal thinking and are sometimes part of a mental illness, such as the manic symptom of grandiosity, can be difficult to rate or code accurately. The authors also point out that children are suggestible and the mere mention of a symptom may elicit a positive response. This carefully done study is an important reminder that false positives are a constant threat to the accuracy of psychiatric studies and that pediatric bipolar disorder studies might be particularly vulnerable to them.

Most studies of pediatric bipolar disorder used the K-SADS. This semistructured interview seemed to provide a golden road to error-free psychiatric assessment. The questions in the interview were prepared with exceptional care and repeatedly studied to insure good statistical properties for inclusion in the interview. Nonetheless, the decision as to how a response should be interpreted is left to the interviewer; the diagnosis reached at the end of the interview might reside as much in the mind of the interviewer as in the clinical state of the patient.

Over time there has been variation in the interviews used and in how the pediatric bipolar diagnostic criteria were defined in research studies. As Gabrielle Carlson, MD, of the New York State University at Stony Brook Medical School has noted, "At present, ironically, we have a situation that did not develop purposely and that really was not recognized until recently. That is, although each research group uses usually one form or another of the K-SADS, and all use *DSM-IV* criteria, different research groups have diverged somewhat in how the interviews are used, what kinds of questions are asked, whether criteria are modified, (and, thus, what kinds of responses are counted), and what informants are used" (Carlson and Glovinsky, 2009, p. 266). All of these alterations can change how the disorder is diagnosed.

MIXING APPLES AND ORANGES

Another little-discussed methodological problem with most of the studies of pediatric bipolar disorder is that children and adolescents are combined. Most of the studies included prepubertal and postpubertal subjects without giving a breakdown by age. The results are not grouped by age, so there is no way of knowing the number of children 12 and under in the study, their response to medication, or any additional characteristics of the 12 and under children in the studies of this disorder. Children and adolescents are combined in the studies as if there were no difference between them. As it is already accepted that some adolescents meet full *DSM-IV* criteria for bipolar disorder, the controversial question of the existence of pediatric bipolar disorder in children under the age of 12 is not addressed when adolescents and children are combined.

CHICKEN OR EGG?

Other facets of pediatric bipolar disorder seem exempt from the usual technical care given to medical research. In a small but very influential study of stimulant medication and the onset of bipolar disorder, DelBello and colleagues may have played a role in the development of a misconception that has likely had an adverse effect on children diagnosed with ADHD and bipolar disorder (DelBello et al., 2001). Thirty-four adolescents diagnosed with bipolar disorder were studied by DelBello and colleagues to learn which adolescents had ADHD and which adolescents were treated with stimulants. Twenty-one adolescents had been treated with stimulants and 13 had not. The 21 adolescents who had been treated with stimulants had been diagnosed with bipolar disorder at an earlier age (10.7 years) than those who had not been treated with stimulants (13.9 years). The authors conclude that the stimulants may have sensitized the patients to develop bipolar disorder.

This is one interpretation of the data but not the most likely explanation. The most likely explanation of the data is that adolescents who had received stimulants received them because they were more ill to start with. In other words, the illness came first, which was followed by the stimulants—not the other way around. This obvious explanation is not mentioned in the discussion section of the article. Instead, the authors emphasize the possibility that the stimulants sensitized the brains of the patients to develop bipolar disorder. This unwarranted conclusion may have contributed to many psychiatric clinicians' unnecessarily withholding stimulant medications for children diagnosed with bipolar disorder and ADHD. As will be described in the next chapter, it has subsequently been repeatedly shown that stimulants can and should be given to children diagnosed with bipolar disorder and ADHD with the promise of great benefit and little risk.

CONCLUSION

There are a number of errors in the scientific study of pediatric bipolar disorder, including changing definitions, combining age groups, and failing to set rules for the evidence that would falsify the diagnosis. It is disappointing that the semistructured psychiatric interview, long the gold standard in research assessment, did not better insure against making the wrong diagnosis; using such instruments can no longer serve as a guarantee of validity. Many of the researchers who undertook the study of pediatric bipolar disorder were vulnerable to misperceiving and misinterpreting the symptoms they evaluated. We are left with a diagnosis with little evidence to support it.

REFERENCES

Breslau, N. (1987). Inquiring about the bizarre: False positives in Diagnostic Interview Schedule for Children (DISC) ascertainment of obsessions, compulsions, and psychotic symptoms. *J Am Acad Child Adolesc Psychiatry, 26*(5), 639–644.

Carlson, G. A., & Glovinsky, I. (2009). The concept of bipolar disorder in children: A history of the bipolar controversy. *Child Adolesc Psychiatr Clin N Am, 18*(2), 257–271, vii.

DelBello, M. P., Soutullo, C. A., Hendricks, W., Niemeier, R. T., McElroy, S. L., & Strakowski, S. M. (2001). Prior stimulant treatment in adolescents with bipolar disorder: Association with age at onset. *Bipolar Disord, 3*(2), 53–57.

Ghaemi, S. N., & Martin, A. (2007). Defining the boundaries of childhood bipolar disorder. *Am J Psychiatry, 164*(2), 185–188.

Heclo, H. (2008). *On Thinking Institutionally.* In L. S. Maisel (Ed.), *On Politics,* 5 vols. Boulder, CO: Paradigm.

10

Stimulant Medications

One of the most dramatic, rapid, and safe treatments in modern medicine is stimulant medication for attention deficit hyperactivity disorder (ADHD) (Pliszka, 2007). Giving stimulant medication at the correct dose to a hyperactive, distracted, and rapidly talking child very often results within two hours in a quiet, well-behaved child. Stimulant medications deserve thoughtful consideration in any discussion of pediatric bipolar disorder, as it is well established that 50% to 90% of children given that diagnosis also have ADHD (Geller et al., 2002; Pavuluri et al., 2006; Singh et al., 2006). Some influential advocates of the pediatric bipolar disorder diagnosis have advised that stimulants make bipolar disorder worse and should not be used in this group of children (DelBello et al., 2001; Faedda et al., 2004; Wendling, 2009)—a claim that will be disputed in this chapter. This poor advice often results in preventing children diagnosed with bipolar disorder from receiving the very medication that could improve their symptoms most (McIntyre, 2009).

There is an immense amount of scientific support for stimulants in the treatment of ADHD. Hundreds of studies have reported success in the short-term stimulant treatment of this disorder (McIntyre, 2009; Pliszka, 2007; National Institutes of Health Consensus Development Conference Statement: Diagnosis and Treatment of Attention-Deficit/ Hyperactivity Disorder [ADHD], 2000; Practice Parameter for the Use of Stimulant Medications in the Treatment of Children, Adolescents, and Adults, 2002). For the many children who respond well to the medication, the dramatic improvement in symptoms allows for success where there was failure and praise where there was criticism. These children begin to think of themselves in a more positive light. Instead of finding themselves constantly in trouble for their behavior by parents and school authorities, the children discover that they can avoid rule breaking and the poor regard of adults as well as being able to concentrate better and get along with other children in the family and classroom.

An illustration of the value that children place on the improvement in their behavior is the case of Charlie, an eight-year-old boy with severe ADHD. About a month after starting his first stimulant medication, with an excellent result, the development of a side effect made it necessary to switch to another stimulant medication. When faced with the loss of the first stimulant, to the parents' surprise, Charlie began to cry in the family session. He asked, "Does this mean I'll have to be a bad boy again? I don't want to be in trouble all the time again."

Receiving praise for behavior can be a powerful new experience for a child and can change the child's self-view from negative to positive. The importance of this to the child may not always be understood or fully appreciated.

It is widely accepted that stimulants are very effective for ADHD symptoms such as short attention span, difficulty concentrating, impulsivity, and hyperactivity; it is less often appreciated that stimulants are also effective in treating aggression (Connor et al., 2002; Hinshaw, 1991; Kaplan et al., 1990). Aggression is not a *DSM-IV* symptom of ADHD, but it frequently accompanies it. Aggression occurs often in oppositional defiant disorder, which is frequently diagnosed along with ADHD. Reduction of aggression is an important bonus in the use of stimulants for the treatment of the children with whom this book is primarily concerned: very angry children with ADHD. It is not in the best interest of these children to give them a diagnosis of bipolar disorder and then withhold stimulant medication because of the false belief that stimulants will worsen this condition.

ETHICAL CONSIDERATIONS

Sometimes the very effectiveness of stimulant medication creates alarm. To many people, it may not seem quite right or ethical to use a medication to stop what is seen as a child's misbehavior; dramatically changing a child's behavior simply by giving a pill is disturbing. The underlying belief is that the child does not have an illness, and medication would be unnecessary if parents were more involved in their children's lives and disciplined them more effectively or if teachers kept order in the classroom. Stimulant medication is seen as providing a convenient way to evade responsibilities rather than an appropriate and needed medical treatment for a disabling illness. Although, as will be discussed later in this chapter, parent or teacher interventions are rarely effective in the absence of medication, the beliefs persist that there is something distasteful about the treatment of ADHD with stimulant medication.

The success of stimulant medications also underscores the belief—or fear—that behavior and personality are shaped by biological forces that can be manipulated. For some, this may almost seem to challenge the notion of free will. In my experience, many parents who hold these views come to appreciate the role of medication and feel reassured about it once they have a chance to see its effects in their own child. As the parents of the successfully stimulant treated ADHD child gain experience with the medication, they become personally acquainted with the medication's strengths and limitations in their child and the medication appears less mysterious and threatening. Also, with their doctor's advice and help, they gain experience in the management of side effects the medication may cause and develop a sense of competence about the use of the medication.

A common fear expressed by parents is that their "real" child will be lost; they fear that their child's unique "spark" or personality will be blunted or lessened by the use of the medication. In my experience, however, the opposite is more often the case. The parents of the appropriately medicated child come to realize that the child is actually *more* like himself or herself—the child is able to more happily and actively engage with the world, and the parents and child are able to get through the day without endless skirmishes about such things as homework or forgotten chores.

Another implicit ethical concern in the use of stimulant medication is the value of suffering in the child's life. In the debates about medication, this concern has been described as "psychopharmacological Puritanism." In this view, ADHD is seen as an obstacle, and overcoming obstacles is seen as being of value for the child's character development. This puritanical attitude is most clearly expressed by some fathers of ADHD boys who complain, "I had the same problem as a child and I didn't take any medicine. I did all right, and he can do all right, too." Absent from such discussions are the distinct possibilities that the father may have done better had he been medicated, or that the child may not be able to overcome the obstacle as well as the father did and instead the ADHD handicap may hinder the child's academic performance, ability to form friendships, job choice, and many other important areas of functioning.

In part, the disdain for stimulant medication for children also may stem from distaste for the large amount of money made by the pharmaceutical industry. Here the assumption seems to be that these companies are pushing the medications on doctors and patients in an effort to turn a bigger profit. In a capitalistic society, such as ours, all goods and services are developed, purchased, and sold with the understanding that a profit for someone is involved. Whether the profit is disproportionate to the value of the product is a legitimate question, but it does not bear directly on the medications' effectiveness, the amount of symptom reduction gained by their use, or the potential benefits they may create in children's lives.

Objections to stimulant medications have been noted and supported by mainstream media, which in turn have had an enormous effect on popular opinion. The *New York Times* has run articles that suggest it is better to treat ADHD with psychotherapy and no medication (Carey, 2006; Parker-Pope, 2008)

The dislike for treating childhood psychiatric illness with drugs, and stimulant drugs in particular, appears to unite the political left and right in this country. On the HBO political comedic talk show *Real Time with Bill Maher* on August 7, 2009, the show's host—an outspoken liberal—invited three guests to discuss the subject—Arianna Huffington, a liberal blogger (huffingtonpost.com), and two conservative congressmen: Rep. Jack Kingston (R-GA) and Rep. Darrell Issa (R-CA). All agreed that psychiatric drugs for children were deplorable. One of the conservative congressmen believed that the problem of misbehaving children might be solved by spanking. Ms. Huffington disliked the spanking idea but felt that medications for children were overused and largely unnecessary. Unusual for this program, a dissenting point of view was not heard.

Objections to medications are understandable; no one wants to see a child medicated if it is not absolutely necessary. But the objections also seem largely to miss the point that these children, and their families, are suffering from an actual illness with clearly defined symptoms and that the most successful treatments include medication. It is doubtful that the same sentiments would be voiced if the medication were for a condition widely understood to be physical such as diabetes or asthma. Treating an ADHD child with the proper medication at the proper dosage can dramatically improve the quality of life for the child.

INCREASE OF USE IN STIMULANT MEDICATION

Closely related to these ethical concerns is the concern over the apparent increase in the use of stimulant medication in the last two decades. At times, the press has alarmed the public by suggesting a vast overuse of stimulants—even creating visions of railroad freight cars trundling across the nation at night filled to the top with stimulants (Hancock, 1996; Schmidt, 1987). A closer examination of relevant research and statistics is reassuring.

The fact that stimulant use has increased is indisputable. Although there is some variation in the statistics reported, there was a marked increase in the use of stimulant medication throughout the eighties and nineties (Safer, Zito, & Fine, 1996). In 1987 the percent of children 18 and younger taking stimulants for ADHD was 0.6%; by 1997 that number had risen to 2.4%, an increase of roughly 400% (Olfson et al., 2002).

In the late 1990s the rate of increase of stimulant use seemed to have leveled off. For example, a major national study found that in 1997 the percent of children under the age of 19 was 2.7%, and by 2002 it was 2.9% (Zuvekas, Vitiello, & Norquist, 2006). This was understood as evidence of a slight overall increase. In adolescents the rate of the use of stimulants continues to increase (Swanson & Volkow, 2009; Visser & Lesesne, 2005; Zuvekas, Vitiello, & Norquist, 2006); it is more widely appreciated that many adolescents continue to have ADHD and that it often does not end by age 12. Also, adolescents use stimulants as drugs of abuse or for weight loss rather than for the medical treatment of symptoms of ADHD (Poulin, 2001).

Of greater importance from a clinical perspective is whether stimulant medication is underprescribed to children who do have ADHD or overprescribed to children who do not have ADHD. An examination of carefully collected data about rates of diagnosis and stimulant use supports the concern that it is underprescribed.

The Centers for Disease Control National Survey of Children's Health reports a U.S. rate of ADHD among children 17 and younger as 7.7% for 2003 (Pastor & Ruben, 2008). A more conservative estimate is that about 5% of all children have ADHD (Zuvekas, Vitiello, & Norquist, 2006). Even with the more conservative estimate it would appear that stimulant medications may be underprescribed rather than overprescribed, as they are given to fewer than 3% of all children. This would mean that approximately 40% of children with ADHD do not receive stimulant medication.

Supporting this estimate, in a closely related study, the Centers for Disease Control (CDC) found that in 2003 only 56% of the children in the United States with ADHD were receiving medication treatment for ADHD (Visser & Lesesne, 2005).

In a 1999 NIMH study, Peter Jensen, MD, a child psychiatrist and a leader in the NIMH children's branch at the time, sent teams of interviewers to homes in four geographically distinct communities to assess the mental health problems of the children in the family and to learn about the treatments the children were receiving (Jensen et al., 1999). Only 12.5% of the children diagnosed with ADHD were receiving stimulant medication. In this study, once again, the children were undertreated.

My own clinical experience also suggests that stimulant medications are underprescribed, as a considerable portion of my professional workday is devoted to persuading parents to try these medications for their untreated and highly symptomatic children with ADHD.

As an example, consider Arlene, a gregarious, talkative eight-year-old girl who was transferred to a special education setting over her mother's objections. The mother believed that Arlene's former teacher had lied about her behavior in regard to a scuffle Arlene had had with another child at school. The mother also believed the school had misrepresented Arlene's behavior as requiring psychiatric evaluation and possibly medication. She thought placement in the special education setting was a mistake that would stain her daughter's academic career, and wanted her daughter returned to the regular school setting immediately. Once the mother's trust had been gained to some degree, a history of the child's behaviors from age three to the present indicated that the child had long-standing symptoms of ADHD. In the special education setting, again, it quickly became apparent to all that the child was continuing to have great difficulties sitting still, concentrating, and organizing her work. In this case, the mother's distrust of medication was compounded by her distrust of the school system. With a great deal of support, the mother reluctantly consented to a trial of stimulant medication, which quickly and obviously helped her child. The mother and the child were greatly relieved by the child's dramatic improvement, and the child was able to return rapidly to a regular school setting.

I routinely see children who would obviously benefit from stimulant medication but whose parents have been persuaded by their friends and the media that these medications should be avoided at all costs.

THE MTA STUDY

No discussion of stimulant medications can be undertaken without some understanding of the most important study in contemporary child psychiatry, the Multimodal Treatment of ADHD study, also called the MTA study (a 14-month randomized clinical trial of treatment strategies for attention-deficit/hyperactivity disorder) (The MTA Cooperative Group, 1999). This study, which explored the best treatments for ADHD, was conducted by a large group of leading child mental health experts and was funded by the National Institute of Mental Health. It was undertaken in order to learn more about the treatment effects of medication and the role of psychotherapy in the treatment of ADHD. It provided scientific answers to questions that had vexed ADHD clinicians and parents of ADHD children for decades.

Planning for the study began in 1992. At that time most treatment studies of stimulant medications and ADHD had been limited to several weeks. The MTA studied the treatment of ADHD for 14 months. After the 14-month treatment phase of the study was over, the researchers continued to track the children to see how they fared. Papers from the study continue to be published on a regular basis.

In the 14-month study 545 patients with ADHD, combined type (inattentive and hyperactive/impulsive), were drawn from various sources in community settings. The average age at the beginning of the study was 8.5 years, with 80% boys and 20% girls. The group was racially mixed, with 61% white, 20% African American, and 19% Hispanic. In addition to ADHD, the children had a variety of other diagnoses, such as anxiety disorders and oppositional defiant disorder.

The 545 children selected for the study were randomly assigned to one of four treatment groups. The first group was Medication Management. The children in this group were treated only with the short-acting (or "immediate release") stimulant methylphenidate (brand name Ritalin), which works only for four hours and requires dosing throughout the day. Short-acting stimulants were in routine use at the time the study started. The dose of methylphenidate was carefully adjusted (titrated) to ensure that the child received a dose that achieved maximal symptom improvement. During this four-week titration phase the dose fluctuated daily and raters who did not know the dose rated the patients' behavior daily (Greenhill et al., 1996).

The medication was given three times a day. After the titration period had established the optimal dose, the children were seen by a child psychiatrist once a month for 30 minutes and there was a brief phone conference between the treating psychiatrist and the classroom teacher before each monthly visit.

The second group received Behavioral Treatment. This included an elaborate behavioral program designed to help the child with ADHD and other difficulties. The parents of the children attended 35 sessions of instruction in behavioral management techniques. The children attended daily full-day sessions at a summer treatment program for 8 weeks. Afterwards, the study placed a behavioral aide in the classroom for 12 weeks. The aide was supervised by the social worker who had been meeting with the parents and who worked with the child over the 8-week summer camp. The children in the Behavioral Treatment group did not receive any stimulant medication.

The third group was the Combination Treatment group. This group received both the medication as delivered in the Medication Management group and the behavioral program of the Behavioral Treatment group. Efforts were made to integrate the two treatment programs to allow the psychiatrist who prescribed the medication to meet with the behavioral therapist on a regular basis.

Also included in the study was a fourth group, the Community Care group. Members of this group were allowed to choose a community ADHD care provider so as to receive the care that would have been provided if the child had not been in the study. This was done in order to compare the three studied treatments to "usual care"—what a family seeking treatment would ordinarily do if they weren't in the study. The parents could choose pediatricians, psychiatrists, psychologists, or counselors and were free to choose or not choose to have their child receive medication. The children in the Community Care group were evaluated regularly by the research project staff. Slightly more than two-thirds (68%) of the children in this group were prescribed stimulant medication by their community care provider.

Which group did the best? At the conclusion of the study, after 14 months, stimulant medication was the clear winner for the treatment of symptoms of ADHD. The greatest improvement in ADHD symptoms occurred for the Medication Management group (medication alone) and the Combination Treatment group (medication with behavior therapy). These two groups were about the same in effectiveness. The Behavioral Treatment and Community Care groups were about the same as each other and dramatically less effective than the Medication Management and Combination Treatment groups. In fact, about one-third of the children in the Behavioral Treatment group had to be given medication for their ADHD during the 14-month study because of the severity of their symptoms. After the 14-month study an additional 25% of the Behavioral Treatment group opted to use medication. The MTA study suggested that psychotherapy without medication for ADHD, even in its most intensive and sophisticated form, was not the best treatment for ADHD.

A comparison of the Community Care group with the Medication Management and Combination Treatment groups provides invaluable information about how ADHD patients should be treated with stimulant medication. Recall that the Community Care group was sent to practitioners in the community to receive care as usually given in the community; there were no study-provided guidelines for community practitioners to follow. Roughly two-thirds (68%) of the Community

Care subjects were given stimulant medication, but these children did poorly in comparison to the Medication Management and Combination Treatment groups. The reason for this was that the Community Care doctors gave the medication differently from the study doctors.

First, the Community Care children on medication were only seen twice a year by the medication-dispensing physician; the children in the Medication Management and Combination Treatment groups were seen once a month by study physicians. Second, the Community Care children were given their medication twice a day, compared to three times a day for the children in the Medication Management and Combination Treatment study groups. Third, the Community Care children did not have the dose of medication titrated (adjusted gradually until an optimal dose is reached) as did the children in the Medication Management and Combination Treatment study groups. Fourth, the Community Care group gave lower doses of medication than did the Medication Management and Combination Treatment groups. Finally, unlike the study physicians for the Medication Management and Combination Treatment study groups, the Community Care group physicians did not receive information from the school about the severity of the child's symptoms or response to medication (Jensen et al., 2001; Murray et al., 2008).

At the time of the MTA study there were no widely used long-acting stimulants. Currently, there are many on the market. The two most frequently used, methylphenidate extended release (brand name, Concerta) and mixed amphetamine salts extended release (brand name, Adderall XR), mimic the three doses per day of the short-acting stimulant. This is based in part on the obvious superiority of the Medication Management and Combination groups' prescription strategy (short-acting stimulants three times per day) as compared to the Community Care group's prescription strategy (short-acting stimulants two times per day) as shown in the MTA study.

Overall, what this study showed was that properly administered stimulants were a highly effective treatment for ADHD over the 14-month period of the study, that the most effective way to give short-acting stimulants was three times a day at an adequate dose and supervised at least monthly by a physician, and that even exceptionally comprehensive behavioral treatment alone was much less effective than stimulants for ADHD.

The Combination Treatment group, which combined behavioral approaches with medication, did provide more benefit to children with ADHD who were also anxious and oppositional. Such children had less anxiety and oppositionality after Combination Treatment than after Medication Management treatment alone. Also, for all ADHD children, the parents in the Combination Treatment group became more effective at managing their children. Those parents whose children were in the Behavioral Treatment group without medication continued to have difficulties with their children. Children in the Combination Treatment group required 20% less medicine at the end of the 14-month period of the study than children in the Medication Management group (Vitiello et al., 2001).

Contributing to the singular importance of the MTA study are the regular follow-up studies of the participants. Recall that after the 14 months of the four treatment groups, the parents were free to obtain any treatment they wished for their children. The study continued to make observations of the children's behavior with the parents' permission.

The most recent follow-up of participants in the original MTA study tells us a considerable amount about the fate of patients with ADHD. This follow-up took place eight years after the 14-month control study ended, when the children were 13 to 18 years of age (Molina et al., 2009). About one-third of those originally on stimulant medication remained on stimulant medication, although this was defined simply as having taken the medication more than 50% of the time. The medication was given by a community provider, a method that had already been demonstrated to be inadequate in the 14-month study. Perhaps these reasons are why the differences apparent at the end of the initial period of controlled treatment were not visible six to eight years later; there was no difference in the symptoms of the adolescents based on the group to which they had been assigned during the 14-month treatment control study.

A comparison group of classmate peers without ADHD had begun to be followed two years after the 14-month study ended to compare with the original ADHD-study children. Several years later, this comparison group performed on average at a much higher level on a variety of measures than did the ADHD-study children. The crucial issue, as yet unknown, is whether the children who had participated in the study, given adequate medication treatment over the eight-year follow-up period, would have performed at a level approximating that of the normal non-ADHD comparison group.

Also of importance, considering the claim that stimulants "cause" or "precipitate" or "exacerbate" pediatric bipolar disorder, is that none of the children in the MTA sample were found at the eight-year follow-up to have a diagnosis of bipolar disorder. The most frequent diagnosis in the eight-year follow-up was conduct disorder or delinquency. The MTA authors concluded that there was no evidence that stimulants led to bipolar disorder in children with ADHD (Molina et al., 2009).

STIMULANT RISKS

Stimulant medication has some well-recognized initial side effects; appetite suppression and sleep difficulty are two of the most common, and both are easily managed. The MTA study provided an opportunity to examine whether stimulants might have more serious long-term side effects, which continues to be a topic for serious scientific study.

Weight and height. For a long time it had been debated whether stimulants decreased the rate of growth and whether children who took them would end up shorter as adults. Safer and colleagues were the first to report that stimulants slowed increases in height and weight and offered the hypothesis that children caught up with respect to height and weight after stopping the medication (Safer, Allen, & Barr, 1975). In 1992, at the time the MTA study was planned, it was generally believed that stimulants had no substantial permanent effect on growth or weight; thus there were no plans to study this at the initiation of the MTA study.

As part of the analysis of data after the third year of the study, however, weight and height were examined. To the surprise of many, when the height and weight of children with ADHD entering the MTA study who had never been treated with stimulants were compared to the height and weight of children their age on standard height and weight tables, it was found that children with ADHD were taller and weighed more. This finding was unexpected (Swanson et al., 2007).

At the six- to eight-year follow-up, the children who took stimulants regularly had grown less than the children who had not taken stimulants regularly. This finding has been repeated in other studies, and today it is generally accepted that there is an overall effect on height—up to about one inch—for continued use of stimulants over several years (Faraone et al., 2008).

In part because of this side effect, many physicians give "stimulant holidays" (weekends or even summer vacations off stimulants) for children whose behavior is not too disruptive. Some families choose to have their children avoid stimulants entirely because of a fear of a possible long-term loss of height. Families must weigh the cost of the possibility of up to an inch loss in height compared to the psychological cost of untreated ADHD. Almost always, families elect a trial of stimulant medication, though there are exceptions, such as the case of Adam.

Adam was a tall, thin, 11-year-old boy with ADHD who had been playing basketball since age 8 and was a gifted player. Adam and his parents strongly believed he would have a career in professional basketball, and an inch in height was a priceless commodity for them.

They elected to avoid medication for the treatment of his ADHD, even when nonstimulant medication was offered. He continued to display obvious symptoms of ADHD and poor academic performance.

Heart rate and blood pressure. Stimulant medication does have slight effects on the normal child's heart: it raises the heart rate two to three beats per minute and raises the child's blood pressure one to four mm mercury (a barely detectable amount with a standard blood pressure cuff) (Gutgesell et al., 1999). Though these small changes have no known immediate ill effects on the normal heart, they may have contributed to a long-standing suspicion that stimulant medication might be related to sudden unexplained death in childhood.

Sudden unexplained death with stimulant medication. Although not widely appreciated, there is a rare but persistent rate of sudden unexplained death in children and adolescents on no medication. The American Academy of Pediatrics reports that the rate of sudden unexplained death in the entire population of children and adolescents is estimated at 8 to 62 per million (Perrin, Friedman, & Knilans, 2008). In children and adolescents taking stimulants it is approximately two per million (Perrin, Friedman, & Knilans, 2008). Even though the statistics reported by the American Academy of Pediatrics suggest that children and adolescents on stimulants may have less chance of sudden unexplained death than children and adolescents not on stimulants, the suspicion lingers that stimulants are associated with sudden unexplained death.

The study of the possible relationship between stimulant medication and sudden unexplained death in childhood led to one of the more bizarre episodes in the contemporary interaction between the Food and Drug Administration and the professional societies of child psychiatry, pediatrics, and cardiology. Kenneth Towbin, MD, a child psychiatrist, has brought much needed clarity to the episode in an editorial in the *Journal of the American Academy of Child and Adolescent Psychiatry* (Towbin, 2008).

As described by Dr. Towbin, in February 2006, the FDA called a meeting of a group called the Drug Safety and Risk Management Advisory Committee (DSaRM). The committee was asked to develop research strategies to study the cardiac risks of stimulant medications (U.S. Department of Health and Human Services, 2006). During the meeting, Dr. Nissen, a distinguished adult cardiologist who did not see or treat children with ADHD, complained that stimulants were overprescribed. He believed overprescription could be reduced by "putting some roadblocks" into the prescription of these medications by calling attention to their "cardiovascular implications." By a narrow margin, the committee called for a special warning at the beginning of the prescribing information for physicians (known as a "black box warning") about the cardiac effects of stimulants. Dr. Nissen famously said, "I want to cause people's hands to tremble a little before they write that script," and he felt that a black box warning was the best way to do this (U.S. Department of Health and Human Services, 2006, p. 223). Dr. Nissen wrote an article summarizing his critical views of stimulants and the risk he felt they posed to cardiac function in the prestigious *New England Journal of Medicine* (Nissen, 2006*).*

Pediatricians and child psychiatrists did not agree with Dr. Nissen's recommendations. When the FDA asked a different group, the Pediatric Advisory Committee, to review the recommendations of the first committee, the Pediatric Advisory Committee voted unanimously that a black box warning was unnecessary, and indeed a black box warning was never issued. Subsequently, Dr. Biederman wrote a blistering critique of Nissen, calling attention to Dr. Nissen's lack of factual knowledge about ADHD and its treatment with stimulants (Biederman et al., 2006).

At about the same time, the American Heart Association seemed to recommend that electrocardiograms (ECGs) be given to all children before they begin stimulant medications. (Gutgesell et al., 1999). The American Academy of Child and Adolescent Psychiatry declined to endorse this recommendation. The American Academy of Pediatrics bluntly rejected it: "A recommendation to obtain ECGs for children receiving ADHD medications is not warranted" (Perrin, Friedman, & Knilans, 2008, p. 452). In September 2008, the American Heart Association softened its recommendation by leaving the decision to obtain an ECG up to the judgment of the physician (Vetter et al., 2008).

Today, an ECG is not usually obtained prior to giving stimulant medication, and the risks associated with the slight raise in heart rate and blood pressure are deemed acceptable by most physicians. If the child has a heart problem or if family members have heart problems an ECG is recommended (Vetter et al., 2008).

Social withdrawal and emotional constriction. Infrequent side effects that occupy a prominent place in the public perception of stimulant medication are social withdrawal and emotional constriction. As discussed on the PBS television program, *Frontline* (September 11, 2000), parents may be afraid their children will become "zombie-like," lose interest in their friends, and lose their spontaneity.

Consider James, a seven-year-old first-grade student. James enjoyed playing with his many friends and was seen as creative and bright. Despite these desirable qualities, officials from James' school called his mother several times a week to report that James was disrupting the class by loudly talking, leaving his seat, and refusing to follow directions. After an evaluation, the diagnosis of ADHD was made, and James was begun on stimulant medication. His behavior and grades improved dramatically, and he even won awards for "most improved" student at the end of first grade. His improved behavior continued through the second grade and half of the third grade. In the middle of third grade, his teachers and mother noted that he seemed suddenly withdrawn, preoccupied, and uninterested in his friends and family members. Neither they nor he could provide a reason to account for this. His stimulant medication was switched from one stimulant to another, and his constricted behavior immediately improved. While maintaining his improvement in his ADHD, he resumed happily playing with his friends and interacting with his family.

Another example is Keisha, a gifted 10-year-old girl who was intensely hyperactive, distractible, and talkative at home and school. On a low dose of stimulant medication her symptoms of ADHD disappeared. Also, she was calmer and much more able to engage in conversations with friends and family. She said, "I feel more mature, but the medicine ruined my creativity." Before the stimulant medication she had loved writing and had written many pages of stories and some poetry each week. She no longer had an urge to do this and had stopped writing completely. "Writing was the only way I could calm myself, but with the medicine keeping me calm, I just don't feel like writing anymore." A change in stimulant medication and support from the family for her writing efforts led to a full resumption of her writing activities and their attendant pleasure while maintaining her complete ADHD improvement.

It is the task of the physician to prescribe medication such that the child achieves the treatment benefits while retaining the child's exuberance and joyful engagement with the world. The identity of the child becomes one of a child with ADHD who can control his or her symptoms on medication and becomes symptomatic off medication. Matter-of-fact acceptance of this situation is an important psychological treatment goal for the child and family. Knowing that there is a medication that is helpful and enables better behavior and school performance should come to be understood as a source of strength and reassurance for the child. Most social side effects or emotional constriction are easily managed with a change of dose or a change of stimulant medication.

Illicit use of stimulants. A natural concern for some parents is the fear that the therapeutic use of stimulants in childhood might lead to drug abuse later in life. Stimulants are considered potential drugs of abuse by the FDA and require a special prescription. The studies in this area are somewhat ambiguous, but several issues seem clear. First, stimulants prescribed by a physician and taken as prescribed do not cause euphoria (feeling high), cravings for more medication, or withdrawal. Second, there is no evidence of addiction to stimulants when they are prescribed by a physician and taken during childhood.

What makes the situation less clear is that a major long-term outcome of childhood ADHD is conduct disorder or delinquency. In the MTA study 25% of the children in the original 14-month study became delinquent or developed a conduct disorder during adolescence (Molina et al., 2007). Delinquency is associated with a high rate of drug abuse, and those children with ADHD who become delinquents will abuse drugs and alcohol at a relatively high rate regardless of whether they took stimulants as children.

Earlier studies of the drug abuse problem found that children who were treated with stimulants for ADHD actually were *less* likely to abuse drugs in later years than those with ADHD who were not treated with stimulants (Wilens, 2004; Wilens et al., 2003). Unfortunately, more recent studies of stimulant treatment during childhood and substance abuse during adolescence do not confirm the protective effect of stimulant treatment with regard to drug abuse. The view held at the moment is that treating ADHD with stimulants during childhood provides neither a protective effect nor an increased risk for developing substance abuse during adolescence or later in life (Biederman, Monuteaux et al., 2008; Biederman, Petty et al., 2008; Mannuzza et al., 2008; Volkow & Swanson, 2008).

There is some evidence that stimulants can be diverted (given to others) at the time they are prescribed. For example, Jennifer Setlik, MD, and colleagues found that when prescription rates for stimulants for adolescents increased, there was a significant increase in calls to poison control centers for stimulant abuse (Setlik, Bond, & Ho, 2009). Another study of 7th to 12th grade students in a survey found that 27% of girls prescribed stimulants and 17% of boys prescribed stimulants reported giving the medication away to their friends (Boyd et al., 2007).

My clinical experience in treating delinquent substance-abusing adolescents for ADHD with stimulants is that it is very difficult to get these adolescents to take the stimulant medication. They do not like the feeling they get from the medication, and they have little interest in improving their academic performance.

Though the abuse of prescribed stimulant medications is a valid concern (more so, it seems, for those who do not need them than for those who do), the fact that these drugs can be abused does not lessen their effectiveness as a treatment for ADHD. For our purposes it seems sufficient to say that the use of stimulants among school-aged children does not seem to have an effect on their later development of drug problems.

Do stimulants make the symptoms of pediatric bipolar disorder worse? As has been mentioned, one of the unfortunate consequences of diagnosing children who do not have bipolar disorder as having bipolar disorder is the withholding of stimulants for the treatment of their ADHD. The belief that stimulants make pediatric bipolar disorder worse led to the prohibition of stimulants for the treatment of the ADHD that so often accompanies the pediatric bipolar disorder diagnosis. This is especially unfortunate as up to 90 percent of children given the diagnosis of pediatric bipolar disorder are also given the diagnosis of ADHD (Singh et al., 2006). Insisting that these children not be treated with stimulant medication has deprived them of the very treatment they most need.

Acceptance of the unsupported belief that stimulant medication may lead to bipolar disorder may have come from the observation that antidepressants may precipitate sudden episodes of acute mania in adolescents and adults predisposed to bipolar disorder (Stoll et al., 1994). In general it is accepted that antidepressants can serve as a precipitant to mania. The inference that stimulant medication can precipitate mania is unwarranted.

Studies have noted that children diagnosed as having pediatric bipolar disorder often had a history of having been prescribed "antidepressants and/or stimulants" prior to the onset of their apparent bipolar disorder symptoms (DelBello et al., 2001; Faedda et al., 2004; Geller, Fox, & Clark, 1994). Taking "antidepressants and/or stimulants" was speculated to have played a causal role in the onset of the disorder or to have made the disorder worse. For example, Ginna Faedda, MD, a child psychiatrist, and her colleagues reviewed the records of 82 children with an average age of 10.6 years who had been diagnosed as having pediatric bipolar disorder. They found that a large proportion of the children had taken a stimulant or an antidepressant in the month before their symptoms were reported to have worsened (Faedda et al., 2004). It is not surprising that patients who are beginning to do poorly might have a trial of medications to learn if the medications might be helpful. This does not mean that the medications caused the so-called bipolar disorder that then followed. Unfortunately, this study and other studies with similarly tentative results left an indelible impression on the field.

Fortunately, substantial evidence has been gathered that stimulants can be safely given to children diagnosed with pediatric bipolar disorder (Carlson et al., 2000; Findling et al., 2007). Of particular interest is a study by Galanter and colleagues in which data from the first month of the MTA study were reanalyzed (Galanter et al., 2005). It will be recalled that the children in the Medication Management group of the

MTA study all received stimulant medication in doses high enough to relieve their ADHD symptoms. Dr. Galanter and colleagues divided the Medication Management group into those patients with symptoms similar to symptoms of bipolar disorder and those without such symptoms. The Galanter group found that there was no difference in the two groups' responses to stimulant medication. There were also no side effects suggesting the onset or worsening of bipolar disorder in either group. In other words, the two groups of children responded exactly the same to the stimulant medication, and neither group developed bipolar-like symptoms as the result of the stimulant medication.

This finding was corroborated in an exceptionally careful study (Waxmonsky et al., 2008) in which 101 children participated in a Summer Treatment Program for children with ADHD. This study, called the Summer Treatment Program study, seems to provide a definitive answer to the question of whether stimulants worsen pediatric bipolar disorder. It also provides strong evidence for the thesis of this book: that most so-called pediatric bipolar disorder is instead a severe form of ADHD and Oppositional Defiant Disorder (ODD).

The Summer Treatment Program met nine hours per day, five days per week, and lasted for nine weeks. In addition to their ADHD, 33 of the 101 children had symptoms such as tantrums and rage that have been called pediatric bipolar disorder and have been recently termed "severe mood dysregulation" or "SMD" (Leibenluft et al., 2003). Many symptoms were measured including ADHD symptoms, ODD symptoms, and mania symptoms from the Young Mania Rating Scale (YMRS). The children with severe mood dysregulation had higher YMRS scores than the children with ADHD+ODD. All children in the program had ADHD: 72% of the SMD children had ODD and 46% of the children without SMD had ODD.

The Summer Treatment Program administered varying doses of the common short-acting stimulant methylphenidate (Ritalin) along with behavior modification to the ADHD+severe mood dysregulation children and to the ADHD+ODD children throughout the nine-week program. The staff, parents, and children did not know what dose was being given, and the staff who rated ADHD symptoms did know whether the children were in the ADHD+severe mood dysregulation group or the ADHD+ODD group. The Summer Treatment Program study found that methylphenidate plus behavior modification was very helpful to both the ADHD+severe mood dysregulation children and the ADHD+ODD children. In both groups, the symptoms of ADHD and ODD improved greatly. Aggression decreased in both groups. Importantly, even symptoms of mania decreased in the ADHD+severe mood dysregulation group. The YMRS decreased by 34%. In addition, so-called core symptoms of pediatric bipolar disorder, as defined by the Geller group, such as elevated mood, also improved.

The Summer Treatment Program study provides scientific support, using a rigorous experimental design, for some of the main theses in this book. First, the authors of the study note that the lack of differences in treatment response between the two groups suggests that the ADHD+severe mood dysregulation group was just a more severe form of the ADHD and ODD spectrum rather than a separate diagnosis of bipolar disorder. Second, the study indicates that even if one were to accept the diagnosis of pediatric bipolar disorder, stimulants do not worsen the symptoms associated with that diagnosis. Finally, the study indicates that stimulants were dramatically effective for children who suffer from ODD or severe mood dysregulation symptoms in addition to ADHD.

CONCLUSION

The decision to place a child on stimulant medication is not something to be taken lightly; the same might be said for the decision *not* to do so. For those families who have decided to treat their child's ADHD with stimulant medication, and for those families who are considering this possibility, I hope this chapter has offered some measure of reassurance that these drugs are a safe and effective treatment, provided they are monitored carefully by a qualified physician. They do not exacerbate the symptoms associated with pediatric bipolar disorder and in fact seem to relieve many of them.

REFERENCES

Biederman, J., Monuteaux, M. C, Spencer, T., Wilens, T. E., Macpherson, H. A., & Faraone, S. V. (2008). Stimulant therapy and risk for subsequent substance use disorders in male adults with ADHD: a naturalistic controlled 10-year follow-up study. *Am J Psychiatry, 165*(5), 597–603.

Biederman, J., Petty, C. R., Dolan, C., Hughes, S., Mick E., Monuteaux, M. C, & Faraone, S. V. (2008). The long-term longitudinal course of oppositional defiant disorder and conduct disorder in ADHD boys: Findings from a controlled 10-year prospective longitudinal follow-up study. *Psychol Med, 38*(7), 1027–1036.

Biederman, J., Spencer, T. J., Wilens, T. E., Prince, J. B., & Faraone, S. V. (2006). Treatment of ADHD with stimulant medications: Response to Nissen perspective in the New England Journal of Medicine. *J Am Acad Child Adolesc Psychiatry, 45*(10), 1147–1150.

Boyd, C. J., McCabe, S. E., Cranford, J. A., & Young, A. (2007). Prescription drug abuse and diversion among adolescents in a southeast Michigan school district. *Arch Pediatr Adolesc Med, 161*(3), 276–281.

Carey, B. (2006). Parenting as Therapy for Child's Mental Disorders. *New York Times*, December 22, 2006.

Carlson, G. A., Loney, J., Salisbury, H., Kramer, J. R., & Arthur, C. (2000). Stimulant treatment in young boys with symptoms suggesting childhood mania: a report from a longitudinal study. *J Child Adolesc Psychopharmacol, 10*(3), 175–184.

Connor, D. F., Glatt, S. J., Lopez, I. D., Jackson, D., & Melloni, R. H., Jr. (2002). Psychopharmacology and aggression. I: A meta-analysis of stimulant effects on overt/covert aggression-related behaviors in ADHD. *J Am Acad Child Adolesc Psychiatry, 41*(3), 253–261.

DelBello, M. P., Soutullo, C. A., Hendricks, W., Niemeier, R. T., McElroy, S. L., & Strakowski., S. M. (2001). Prior stimulant treatment in adolescents with bipolar disorder: Association with age at onset. *Bipolar Disord, 3*(2), 53–57.

Faedda, G. L., Baldessarini, R. J., Glovinsky, I. P., & Austin, N. B. (2004). Treatment-emergent mania in pediatric bipolar disorder: A retrospective case review. *J Affect Disord, 82*(1), 149–158.

Faraone, S. V., Biederman, J., Morely, C. P., & Spenser, T. J. (2008). Effect of stimulants on height and weight: A review of the literature. *J. Am. Acad Child Adolesc Psychiatry, 47*.

Findling, R. L., Short, E. J., McNamara, N. K., Demeter, C. A., Stansbrey, R. J., Gracious, B. L., Whipkey, R., Manos, M. J., & Calabrese, J. R. (2007). Methylphenidate in the treatment of children and adolescents with bipolar disorder and attention-deficit/hyperactivity disorder. *J Am Acad Child Adolesc Psychiatry, 46*(11), 1445–1453.

Galanter, C., Pagar, D., Davies, M., Li, W., Carlson, G., Abikoff, H., Arnold, L. E., Bukstein, O., Pelham, W. E., Elliott, G., Hinshaw, S. P., Epstein, J., Wells, K., Hechtman, L., Newcorn, J., Greenhill, L., Wigal, T., Swanson, J., & Jenson, P. (2005). ADHD and manic symptoms: Diagnostic and treatment implications. *Clinical Neuroscience Research, 5*(5), 283–294.

Geller, B., Fox, L. W., & Clark, K. A. (1994). Rate and predictors of prepubertal bipolarity during follow-up of 6- to 12-year-old depressed children. *J Am Acad Child Adolesc Psychiatry, 33*(4), 461–468.

Geller, B., Zimerman, B., Williams, M., DelBello, M. P., Bolhofner, K., Craney, J. L., Frazier, J., Beringer, L., & Nickelsburg, M. J. (2002). DSM-IV mania symptoms in a prepubertal and early adolescent bipolar disorder phenotype compared to attention-deficit hyperactive and normal controls. *J Child Adolesc Psychopharmacol, 12*(1), 11–25.

Greenhill, L. L., Abikoff, H. B., Arnold, L. E., Cantwell, D. P., Conners, C. K., Elliott, G., Hechtman, L., Hinshaw, S. P., Hoza, B., Jensen, P. S., March, J. S., Newcorn, J., Pelham, W. E., Severe, J. B., Swanson, J. M., Vitiello, B., & Wells, K. (1996). Medication treatment strategies in the MTA Study: Relevance to clinicians and researchers. *J Am Acad Child Adolesc Psychiatry, 35*(10), 1304–1313.

Gutgesell, H., Atkins, D., Barst, R., Buck, M., Franklin, W., Humes, R., Ringel, R., Shaddy, R., & Taubert, K. A. (1999). Cardiovascular monitoring of children and adolescents receiving psychotropic drugs: A statement for healthcare professionals from the Committee on Congenital Cardiac Defects, Council on Cardiovascular Disease in the Young, American Heart Association. *Circulation, 99*(7), 979–982.

Hancock, L. (1996, March 18). Mother's little helper. *Newsweek*, 51–56.

Hinshaw, S. P. (1991, September). Stimulant medication and the treatment of aggression in children with attentional deficits. *Journal of Clinical Child Psychology, 20*, 301–312.

Jensen, P.S., Hinshaw, S. P., Swanson, J. M., Greenhill, L. L., Conners, C. K., Arnold, L. E., Abikoff, H. B., Elliott, G., Hechtman, L., Hoza, B., March, J. S., Newcorn, J. H., Severe, J. B., Vitiello, B., Wells, K., & Wigal, T. (2001). Findings from the NIMH Multimodal Treatment Study of ADHD (MTA): Implications and applications for primary care providers. *J Dev Behav Pediatr, 22*(1), 60–73.

Jensen, P.S., Kettle, L., Roper, M.T., Sloan, M.T., Dulcan, M.K., Hoven, C., Bird, H.R., Bauermeister, J.J., & Payne, J.D. (1999). Are stimulants overprescribed? Treatment of ADHD in four U.S. communities. *J Am Acad Child Adolesc Psychiatry, 38*(7), 797–804.

Kaplan, S.L., Busner, J., Kupietz, S., Wassermann, E., & Segal, B. (1990). Effects of methylphenidate on adolescents with aggressive conduct disorder and ADDH: A preliminary report. *J Am Acad Child Adolesc Psychiatry, 29*(5), 719–723.

Leibenluft, E., Charney, D. S., Towbin, K. E., Bhangoo, R. K., & Pine, D. S. (2003). Defining clinical phenotypes of juvenile mania. *Am J Psychiatry, 160*(3), 430–437.

Mannuzza, S., Klein., R. G., Truong, N. L., Moulton, J.L. 3rd, Roizen, E.R., Howell, K.H., & Castellanos, F.X. (2008). Age of methylphenidate treatment initiation in children with ADHD and later substance abuse: Prospective follow-up into adulthood. *Am J Psychiatry, 165*(5), 604–609.

McIntyre, R. (2009). Bipolar disorder and ADHD: Clinical concerns. *CNS Spectr, 14*(7 Suppl 6), 8–9; discussion 13–14.

Molina, B.S., Flory, K., Hinshaw, S. P., Greiner, A. R., Arnold, L. E., Swanson, J. M., Hechtman, L., Jensen, P. S., Vitiello, B., Hoza, B., Pelham, W. E., Elliott, G. R., Wells, K. C., Abikoff, H. B., Gibbons, R. D., Marcus, S., Conners, C. K., Epstein, J. N., Greenhill, L. L., March, J. S., Newcorn, J. H., Severe, J. B., & Wigal, T. (2007). Delinquent behavior and emerging substance use in the MTA at 36 months: Prevalence, course, and treatment effects. *J Am Acad Child Adolesc Psychiatry, 46*(8), 1028–1040.

Molina, B.S., Hinshaw, S. P., Swanson, J. M., Arnold, L. E., Vitiello, B., Jensen, P. S., Epstein, J. N., Hoza, B., Hechtman, L., Abikoff, H. B., Elliott, G. R., Greenhill, L. L., Newcorn, J. H., Wells, K. C., Wigal, T., Gibbons, R. D., Hur, K., & Houck, P. R. (2009). The MTA at 8 years: Prospective follow-up of children treated for combined-type ADHD in a multisite study. *J Am Acad Child Adolesc Psychiatry, 48*(5), 484–500.

The MTA Cooperative Group. Multimodal Treatment Study of Children with ADHD. (1999). Fourteen-month randomized clinical trial of treatment strategies for attention-deficit/hyperactivity disorder. *Arch Gen Psychiatry, 56*(12), 1073–1086.

Murray, D.W., Arnold, L. E., Swanson, J., Wells, K., Burns, K., Jensen, P., Hechtman, L., Paykina, N., Legato, L., & Strauss, T. (2008). A clinical re-view of outcomes of the multimodal treatment study of children with attention-deficit/hyperactivity disorder (MTA). *Curr Psychiatry Rep, 10*(5), 424–431.

National Institutes of Health Consensus Development Conference Statement: Diagnosis and Treatment of Attention-Deficit/Hyperactivity Disorder (ADHD). (2000). *J. Am. Acad. Child Adolesc. Psychiatry, 39*(2), 182–193.

Nissen, S. E. (2006). ADHD drugs and cardiovascular risk. *N Engl J Med, 354*(14), 1445–1448.

Olfson, M., Marcus, S. C., Weissman, M. M., & Jensen, P. S. (2002). National trends in the use of psychotropic medications by children. *J Am Acad Child Adolesc Psychiatry, 41*(5), 514–521.

Parker-Pope, T. (2008). Weighing Nondrug Options for ADHD. *New York Times,* June 17, (2008).

Pastor, P. N., & Reuben, C. A. (2008). Diagnosed attention deficit hyperactivity disorder and learning disability: United States, 2004–2006. National Center for Health Statistics.

Pavuluri, M. N., Schenkel, L. S., Aryal, S., Harral, E. M., Hill, S. K., Herbener, E. S., & Sweeney, J. A. (2006). Neurocognitive function in unmedicated manic and medicated euthymic pediatric bipolar patients. *Am J Psychiatry, 163*(2), 286–293.

Perrin, J. M., Friedman, R. A., & Knilans, T. K. (2008). Cardiovascular monitoring and stimulant drugs for attention-deficit/hyperactivity disorder. *Pediatrics, 122*(2), 451–453.

Pliszka, S. (2007). Practice parameter for the assessment and treatment of children and adolescents with attention-deficit/hyperactivity disorder. *J Am Acad Child Adolesc Psychiatry, 46*(7), 894–921.

Poulin, C. (2001). Medical and nonmedical stimulant use among adolescents: From sanctioned to unsanctioned use. *CMAJ, 165*(8), 1039–1044.

Practice Parameter for the Use of Stimulant Medications in the Treatment of Children, Adolescents, and Adults. (2002). *J. Am. Acad Child Adolesc Psychiatry, 41*(2), 26s–49s.

Safer, D. J., Allen, R. P., & Barr, E. (1975). Growth rebound after termination of stimulant drugs. *J Pediatr, 86*(1), 113–116.

Safer, D. J., Zito, J. M., & Fine, E. M. (1996). Increased methylphenidate usage for attention deficit disorder in the 1990s. *Pediatrics, 98*(6 Pt 1), 1084–1088.

Schmidt, W. E. (1987). Sales of drug are soaring for treatment of hyperactivity. *New York Times,* May 5, 1987.

Setlik, J., Bond, G. R., & Ho, M. (2009). Adolescent Prescription ADHD Medication Abuse Is Rising Along with Prescriptions for These Medications. *Pediatrics, 124*(3), 875–880.

Singh, M. K., Delbello, M. P., Kowatch, R. A., & Strakowski, S. M. (2006). Co-occurrence of bipolar and attention-deficit hyperactivity disorders in children. *Bipolar Disord, 8*(6), 710–720.

Stoll, A. L., Mayer, P. V., Kolbrener, M., Goldstein, E., Suplit, B., Lucier, J., Cohen, B. M., & Tohen, M. (1994). Antidepressant-associated mania: a controlled comparison with spontaneous mania. *Am J Psychiatry, 151*(11), 1642–1645.

Swanson, J. M., Elliott, G. R., Greenhill, L. L., Wigal, T., Arnold, L. E., Vitiello, B., Hechtman, L., Epstein, J. N., Pelham, W. E., Abikoff, H. B., Newcorn, J. H., Molina, B. S., Hinshaw, S. P., Wells, K. C., Hoza, B., Jensen, P. S., Gibbons, R. D., Hur, K., Stehli, A., Davies, M., March, J. S., Conners, C. K., Caron, M., & Volkow, N. D. (2007). Effects of stimulant medication on growth rates across 3 years in the MTA follow-up. *J Am Acad Child Adolesc Psychiatry, 46*(8), 1015–1027.

Swanson, J.M., & Volkow, N.D. (2009). Psychopharmacology: Concepts and opinions about the use of stimulant medications. *J Child Psychol Psychiatry, 50*(1–2), 180–193.

Towbin, K. (2008). Paying attention to stimulants: Height, weight, and cardiovascular monitoring in clinical practice. *J Am Acad Child Adolesc Psychiatry, 47*(9), 977–980.

U.S. Department of Health and Human Services, FDA. Center for Drug Evaluation and Research. (2006). Proceedings of the Drug Safety and Management Advisory Committee Meeting.

Vetter, V.L., Elia, J., Erickson, C., Berger, S., Blum, N., Uzark, K., & Webb, C.L. (2008). Cardiovascular monitoring of children and adolescents with heart disease receiving medications for attention deficit/hyperactivity disorder [corrected]: A scientific statement from the American Heart Association Council on Cardiovascular Disease in the Young Congenital Cardiac Defects Committee and the Council on Cardiovascular Nursing. *Circulation, 117*(18), 2407–2423.

Visser, S. N., & Lesesne, C. A. (2005). Mental Health in the United States: Prevalence of Diagnosis and Medication Treatment for Attention-Deficit/Hyperactivity Disorder—United States, (2003). Edited by C. f. D. C. a. Prevention: Center for Disease Control and Prevention.

Vitiello, B., Severe, J. B., Greenhill, L. L., Arnold, L. E., Abikoff, H. B., Bukstein, O.G., Elliott, G. R., Hechtman, L., Jensen, P. S., Hinshaw, S. P., March, J. S., Newcorn, J. H., Swanson, J. M., & Cantwell, D. P. (2001). Methylphenidate dosage for children with ADHD over time under controlled conditions: Lessons from the MTA. *J Am Acad Child Adolesc Psychiatry, 40*(2), 188–196.

Volkow, N.D., & Swanson, J. M. (2008). Does childhood treatment of ADHD with stimulant medication affect substance abuse in adulthood? *Am J Psychiatry, 165*(5), 553–555.

Waxmonsky, J., Pelham, W. E., Gnagy, E., Cummings, M.R., O'Connor, B., Majumdar, A., Verley, J., Hoffman, M.T., Massetti, G.A., Burrows-MacLean, L., Fabiano, G.A., Waschbusch, D.A., Chacko, A., Arnold, F.W., Walker, K.S., Garefino, A.C., & Robb, J.A. (2008). The efficacy and tolerability of methylphenidate and behavior modification in children with attention-deficit/hyperactivity disorder and severe mood dysregulation. *J Child Adolesc Psychopharmacol, 18*(6), 573–588.

Wendling, P. (2009). Stimulant use in ADHD, bipolar discouraged: Expert in mood disorders cites evidence showing that amphetamines might worsen both ill nesses. *Clinical Psychiatry News*, August 2009.

Wilens, T.E. (2004). Attention-deficit/hyperactivity disorder and the substance use disorders: the nature of the relationship, subtypes at risk, and treatment issues. *Psychiatr Clin North Am, 27*(2), 283–301.

Wilens, T.E., Faraone, S. V., Biederman, J., & Gunawardene, S. (2003). Does stimulant therapy of attention-deficit/hyperactivity disorder beget later substance abuse? A meta-analytic review of the literature. *Pediatrics, 111*(1), 179–185.

Zuvekas, S. H., Vitiello, B., & Norquist, G. S. (2006). Recent trends in stimulant medication use among U.S. children. *Am J Psychiatry, 163*(4), 579–585.

PART III
Advice for Parents

11

Medication Advice
for Parents

This chapter provides some practical tips for parents faced with the recommendation of medication for their children who have been diagnosed with bipolar disorder. As roughly 90% of these children have also been diagnosed with ADHD, the use of stimulant medications will be addressed first. Later the use of antipsychotics in treating aggression will also be discussed.

STIMULANT MEDICATIONS

If your child has been diagnosed with ADHD, your child should almost always be treated with stimulant medication. As discussed in chapter 10, there is strong evidence that stimulant medication makes ADHD better and no good evidence that it makes bipolar disorder worse. There are some children who should not take stimulants (children with certain heart defects and other medical conditions), but this is a rare and should be decided by your doctor.

A lot of parents do not like the idea of having their children take stimulant medication, but the evidence that this is the most effective treatment for ADHD is indisputable. Psychotherapy on its own for ADHD does not work. It may help the children to cope with the disorder to some degree by having them make lists and write down homework assignments, but this is not treatment for the underlying condition.

As a child psychiatrist, one of the saddest things I see is a child with ADHD whose parents have withheld medication treatment throughout elementary school with the misguided belief that this has protected the child. The untreated child with ADHD is vulnerable to developing a pattern of school failure and having chronic behavior problems. Because the child is always in trouble or being scolded the child comes to believe he or she is actually "bad," with resultant loss of self-esteem and the development of a defiant attitude. Having unwittingly established a pattern of school failure and misbehavior throughout the child's elementary school years, the parents all too often first bring their child for treatment in early adolescence after the child's behavior becomes more severe and disruptive. By then, the behavior patterns have been firmly established. Although such adolescents can be helped, it is more difficult and the outcome is less certain than it would have been had the child received earlier treatment.

When the diagnosis is first made, treat your child's ADHD with stimulant medication. The value of the increase in acceptance of peers, family, and school during the elementary school years is incalculable for the child's healthy psychological development.

Stimulant medications may have side effects, as may medications for any illness. Some common stimulant side effects that can usually be managed easily by knowledgeable physicians are sleep difficulties, reduced appetite, and moodiness. Should the child have some medical reason that prevents the use of stimulants, there are alternative medications your doctor can prescribe.

There are many different brands and formulations of stimulant medication on the market, including methylphenidate and dexmethylphenidate (brands include Concerta, Ritalin, Metadate, Focalin, Daytrana Patch), dextroamphetamine and mixed amphetamine salts (brands include Dexedrine, Adderall XR, Vyvanse), and others. I have no preference. In general, the long-acting form of the medication is preferable to the short-acting form of the medication. In the past, children at school lining up at the nurse's office for their lunch time dose of stimulants was a familiar scene. It is largely unnecessary these days as long-acting forms of the medication last throughout the school day. Some children may need a short-acting booster toward the end of the school day because the level of the long-acting stimulant has begun to decline and is no longer effective.

ADHD medications are not given at a fixed dose depending on the age or weight of the child. Rather, the medications must be given at a low dose to start and increased slowly depending on the patient's behavioral response to the medication and side effects. Teacher and parent forms for the child's ADHD symptoms and behavior are critical in assessing how well the medication is working.

Many parents do not realize that stimulant medication only lasts for a day. The medication is effectively out of the body at the end of each day. The medication does not accumulate. Each day it is given it is as if the medication had not been given previously. The medication has a rapid onset of action. In general, its effects are noticeable within one to two hours. Parents should not be concerned if the doctor raises the dose—this does not mean that the child is seriously mentally ill or is not responding as was predicted. It is standard to start at a low dose to make sure the child won't have a serious physical problem from the medication (such as a rare allergic reaction).

Similarly, parents should not be concerned if doses are changed or medications are switched. Parents sometimes are afraid that the doctor is experimenting or using the child patient as a "guinea pig." Parents should be aware that such careful adjustments of doses and changing medications to get the best result are a hallmark of good medical care. There is usually some reason to believe that a group of medications, for example, stimulants, will work for a particular condition, for example, ADHD. But the question of greatest concern—will this particular stimulant work for this particular child—can only be learned by giving the child an adequate dose of a specific stimulant medication for an adequate period of time. The medicine may or may not work and there may or may not be side effects. There is only one way to find out.

There are nonstimulant medications for the treatment of ADHD. In general, they do not work as well as stimulants. Their use is beyond the scope of this book except to note they have an important role in children with whom stimulants cannot be used.

ANTIPSYCHOTIC MEDICATIONS

For very aggressive children, I reluctantly prescribe antipsychotic medications. My reluctance is based upon the risk of undesirable side effects. Use of these medications should be reserved for the most aggressive children. Judicious use of antipsychotic medication for aggression can help prevent children and adolescents from needing to be psychiatrically hospitalized or even placed in juvenile detention centers or some other restrictive form of care outside of the home. The goal of outpatient treatment of extremely aggressive children and adolescents often misdiagnosed as having bipolar disorder is to maintain them in their usual home and school settings.

The term antipsychotic is somewhat of a misnomer for this type of medication. Although the medications are used for the treatment of psychosis and work well for this problem, they are not specific for it. They work exceptionally well for a wide variety of nonpsychotic conditions and are the drug of choice for severe aggression. Although these drugs are reported as working in pediatric bipolar disorder, they are helpful largely because they reduce aggression. Some commonly used SGA antipsychotic medications are aripiprazole (Abilify), olanzapine (Zyprexa), quetiapine (Seroquel), and ziprasidone (Geodon).

Some of the more serious side effects of antipsychotic medications were reviewed in chapter 7, including tardive dyskinesia, akathisia (abnormal amount of restlessness), hormonal changes, neuroleptic malignant syndrome, and excessive weight gain leading to diabetes and other health risks. Patients on antipsychotic medications should be weighed on a monthly basis and examined for the development of stiffness or any muscle or movement changes. A healthy diet and exercise to help avoid weight gain are important, as are periodic laboratory examinations to assess metabolic risk factors.

Some less serious but troublesome side effects of antipsychotic medications include sleepiness, dry mouth, and blurred vision. Most of these side effects can be managed by knowledgeable, attentive physicians.

As with stimulant medications, antipsychotic medications are initially prescribed in low doses and the medication is slowly increased based on the patient's behavioral response and ability to tolerate them.

This brief consideration of side effects of antipsychotic and stimulant medications is not inclusive. All medications come with patient package inserts, which should be kept and referred to for more information. Always discuss any concerns you have with your physician. The risks of taking these medications cannot be dismissed lightly. Taking any medication entails risks, and these medications are no exception. The benefits they can bring are substantial and seem to make the risks worth taking. Working closely with a physician is a necessary condition for minimizing risk.

Given the complexities in the use of stimulant medications and antipsychotic medications, parents may wonder what medication treatment advantage they have gained by not having their child diagnosed as having bipolar disorder. There is indeed a substantial advantage because an appreciation that the child does not have bipolar disorder largely avoids the use of anticonvulsant medications and lithium, which have an array of complications of their own. It also enables the child to receive stimulants, the medication most likely to be helpful yet often withheld.

12

A Family-Based Behavior Modification Program for Oppositional Children

For oppositional and defiant children with ADHD, medication sometimes hits a home run. A defiant, oppositional, unruly, overactive, distractible child who refuses to listen at home and at school might, with medication, quickly become a pleasant cooperative child who begins to achieve in the classroom and win the approval of his parents at home. This happy outcome is occasionally achieved with stimulant medication. More frequently, however, the medication does not hit a home run in these defiant children. It may only get to second or third base. Although the child improves, significant problems often remain. Defiance, anger, and fighting with siblings are among the common behaviors that continue to bedevil the child successfully treated for overactivity and inattention. Behavior modification addresses these leftover problems. It is also useful in other situations; for example, cases in which the parents refuse to allow medication, in which the child is not responsive to medication, or when the child has a medical condition that does not permit the use of medication.

Parents, in their attempts to be helpful to their misbehaving child, will often intuitively turn to some form of behavior modification program; they may try to give rewards for good behavior and try to punish bad behavior. Sometimes this works and the problem behavior is corrected. Often it does not work. It has been my experience that a behavior modification program that has been carefully designed, with clear guidelines and unambiguous consequences that are consistently enforced, has the best chance of success. Having the insight and support of a professional is often helpful to both the parents and the child.

This chapter will describe a simple effective program that therapists and parents can use. The program is first described for therapists and parents. Afterward, a special note for parents only is added.

There are innumerable reasons why a child may not comply with a parent's requests. The child's ADHD may cause the child to be too forgetful or disorganized to comply, and the anxious fearful child may be too afraid to comply. This program is specifically directed to the oppositional defiant child whose refusal to comply is intentional. The program is intended to assist parents in coming together as a team to reassert a benevolent authority in the family and ensure that the child functions with less conflict and higher self-regard.

REINFORCING BAD BEHAVIOR

This program is based on the assumption that oppositional defiant children who misbehave enjoy it on some level and are almost always rewarded by their parents for misbehaving. Of course, most parents don't intend to reward their children for misbehaving, and they are often not aware that this is exactly what they're doing. Over time this habit of bad behavior and inadvertent rewards develops and becomes an entrenched family pattern of interaction. It is therefore helpful to begin a behavior modification program by making it clear to the parents the variety of ways in which they might be inadvertently rewarding the very behavior they are trying to change.

Michael and his parents are good examples. Michael, a 16-year-old boy, hated school and regularly got Ds and Fs despite his demonstrated academic ability. He refused to study and was in constant trouble in school for minor discipline issues. His truculence and defiance at home mirrored his insubordinate behavior at school. He took stimulant medication for ADHD, which helped his hyperactivity and inattention, but his behavior continued to be a problem.

Michael had promised his father he would study, improve his grades, and improve his behavior if only his father bought him his long-desired possession: a motorcycle. The father surrendered to Michael's constant demands with the understanding that Michael would begin to study and improve his behavior after the purchase of the motorcycle. After the bike was purchased Michael continued to refuse to study and remained defiant at school and at home.

Michael's parents had rewarded his misbehavior with a motorcycle. They had a long-standing practice of giving him many material rewards—including video games, DVDs, phones, and a flat-screen cable TV in his bedroom—in the hopes that these would motivate him to change his behavior. Instead, rewarding his misbehavior had ensured that it would persist.

In the majority of cases the rewarding of misbehavior will not be as obvious as this, but the same principle is in operation. I make this clear in a session with the parents and the oppositional child together. I let the family know that although it was not intended, the parents are rewarding the child for misbehaving. I let them know that the child enjoys misbehaving and enjoys getting rewarded for it. I let them know that things will change and the child will instead get rewarded for behaving and not for misbehaving.

Acceptance of the principle that the child is misbehaving because he or she is being rewarded for misbehaving has several constructive consequences. First, it implies that the child has a large element of control over his or her behavior. If the child is behaving in a particular fashion because he or she is rewarded for that behavior, the child may be able to behave differently if the rewards were given differently. Second, it suggests that the parents also have some control over the child's behavior, as they can alter the dynamic so that only good behavior is rewarded.

In addition to addressing the role that parents play in helping to create problem behaviors, it's also crucial at the outset of any behavior modification program to address the child's own contribution. A common dilemma for families and therapists is the "mad versus bad" dilemma, which has at its core the sense of the child's role in his or her behavior—that is, whether or not the child can be held responsible for his or her behavior. A "mad" child misbehaves because the child is mentally ill and should not be held accountable. A "bad" child misbehaves of his or her own free will and should be held accountable. In order for this behavior modification program to work it is helpful to think of the behavior as "bad"—that is, the patient is responsible for his or her behavior. In this way, the family and the patient become active participants in the change process.

Eric and his mother illustrate many of the principles of "mad" versus "bad." Eric was a 10-year-old boy with an explosive temper. Eric constantly demanded a variety of things such as books, toys, and video games from his mother. Angry at his mother after she refused to allow him to listen to a CD, he kicked her and tried to stab her with a pair of scissors. This behavior led to psychiatric hospitalization. In an attempt to apologize to his mother, he told her, "I don't know what comes over me; I just do these things sometimes." His mother had an intense feeling of sympathy for him after hearing his explanation and told me, "I feel so sorry for him; he really can't help it."

In believing that her son couldn't control himself, Eric's mother defined him as "mad" and not responsible for his behavior. From the perspective of the behavior modification program, he is "bad." His behavior was a response to a long history of having his demands immediately met, and it is assumed he had a considerable amount of control over his behavior.

THE BEHAVIOR MODIFICATION PROGRAM: AN OVERVIEW

As listed in Table 12.1, there are four stages of the behavior modification program: Stage I, Rewards List; Stage II, Misbehavior List; Stage III, Baseline Data; and Stage IV, Implementation. A simple description of each stage is provided below. After the four stages have been briefly introduced, each stage will be described in more detail. Finally, aspects of psychotherapy and family therapy of each stage will be discussed. Although the psychotherapy portion of the discussion is directed primarily to therapists, parents are encouraged to read this material to deepen their understanding of the program.

In the first stage, Rewards List, the parents and child together make a list of the child's favorite activities. I encourage them to make the list as long as possible and to include a minimum of 15 favorite activities. We then divide the list into "routine rewards or pleasures" and "special treats." I explain that all of us have simple pleasures that we repeat every day. We repeat them often enough that we might not even notice them as treats or rewards. For example, milk and cookies after school, television, playing outside, and cell phone use are frequent daily rewards the child has come to expect. Coffee the first thing in the morning is used to illustrate a powerful daily reward for parents. I call these "routine rewards."

TABLE 12.1. Behavior Modification Program Stages

1. Stage 1: Rewards List; list routine rewards and special treats; win child over to the program
2. Stage 2: Misbehavior List; list problem behaviors
3. Stage 3: Baseline Data; draw a behavior chart; record number of misbehaviors for each day of one week
4. Stage 4: Implementation;
   2 or less misbehaviors per day = a "good" day—child gets routine rewards and one point for a special treat the next day; four special treat points earns one special treat
   3 misbehaviors a day = an "okay" day—child gets routine rewards the next day, but no points for a special treat
   4 or more misbehaviors per day = a "bad" day—child loses routine rewards the next day and gets no points toward a special treat (but doesn't lose any previously earned special reward points)

"Special treats," by contrast, are special rewards for exceptionally good behavior. Special treats may include a trip to the movies, renting a movie, attending a rock concert, sleeping over at a friend's house, or fishing with a parent. These treats most often take place on a weekend. Patients and their parents usually work on the list of routine rewards and special treats over one or several weeks until the list seems long and comprehensive.

The second stage, Misbehavior List, is usually conducted in a session immediately after the list of routine rewards and special treats has been completed by the family. Again, the parents and child make a list together, this time of the child's misbehaviors. As with the list of rewards and special treats, the family should try to identify as many misbehaviors as possible, with a minimum of 15.

The third stage is Baseline Data. It begins with the parents and child creating a behavior chart. The list of misbehaviors is written down the left margin, and the days of the week are listed across the top of the paper. Over the course of the week a mark is made each time the child displays one of the misbehaviors. This gives a picture of the number of times the child misbehaves each day and the type of behaviors the child displays. The primary purpose of the exercise is to get a week of baseline behaviors before the program is implemented. This chart format is continued during the rest of the program to monitor progress and to keep track of rewards.

If the child only misbehaves three or four times a week, then the program should not be used. It won't work. Frequent behaviors are much easier to change than infrequent behaviors, which are difficult to modify with a behavior modification program.

The fourth and final stage is Implementation, and keeping score is central to this fourth stage. The chart that was used to develop a baseline in the third stage is also used during the Implementation phase. The number of misbehaviors per day is always totaled up at bedtime and then translated into a simple system of rewards and penalties. The rewards and penalties always apply to the *day after*. The actual behavior the day after doesn't affect whether the child gets the rewards or penalties earned the day before.

Two or fewer misbehaviors in a day is considered a "good" day in the program. A child with a good day gets his or her routine rewards the day after, plus a point toward a special treat. Four "good day" points lead to a special treat. The special treat should be awarded as close to earning the treat as possible—ideally on the weekend immediately following the week it was earned. If the child earns four special treat points but misbehaves in some way before spending the points, he or she is still entitled to the special treat and should have it.

Three misbehaviors on a given day is considered an "okay" day. On the day after the okay day, the child may have the routine rewards that were established in the first part of the program. For most children this includes daily activities the child enjoys such as video games, TV, regular bedtime, milk and cookies after school, etc. The child does not earn any special treat points for an okay day.

More than three misbehaviors per day is a "bad" day. On the day after a bad day the child loses all of his or her routine rewards and does not earn any points toward a special treat.

The parents' capacity to implement the deprivations of routine rewards the day following a bad day and the child's capacity to accept these restrictions are the greatest uncertainties of the program. The child may respond with explosive violent behavior, and/or the resolution of the parents may crumble. A bad day can create dread for the parents and resignation or violent defiance for the patient. Managing this potential crisis will be described in more detail below.

Having briefly outlined each stage of the behavior modification program, I will revisit the stages separately to give some tips and advice on how to present each stage to the parent and child. Also, I will consider management of the more difficult aspects of the program more thoroughly.

STAGE I: REWARDS LIST

The first stage, Rewards List, asks the parents, in the presence of the child, to make a list of activities the child enjoys. This is done with the child present in order to keep the program appealing for the child. Often the child has been subjected to long-standing complaints and threats by his or her parents before the treatment. Making a list of rewarding activities for the child immediately shifts the focus of the family discussion and suggests that the child's specific pleasures and wants will be an important focus of the program. The parents stop complaining about the child during the discussion of the rewards list and for a few moments may begin to regard the child more fondly. As this session ends, I often ask the family to continue working on the rewards list during the week before the next session in order to extend the time of the positive interaction between the parent and the child.

In previous paragraphs I have described the child in the program in harsh terms such as "misbehaving" or "enjoying misbehaving." This should not be misunderstood to suggest that the program is tough, hostile, or unfriendly to the child patient. In this session it is particularly important that the child understands that the program is designed to maximize getting rewarded. It is critical to the success of the program that the child is "won over."

This is one reason for demanding that the parents and child come up with a large list of rewarding behaviors. In an effort to persuade the child to support or align himself or herself with the program, I will often say, "It's true you do get rewards from your family, but I don't think you get enough. I want you to get more, and I want you to get them for behaving well instead of behaving badly." The child must believe that there is something for him or her in this program, and this must be accomplished in stage one. Often I begin each session after stage one by asking the family to remind me of the list of special treats and routine rewards. This is done, of course, to remind the family of the pleasurable aspects of the program for the child. Similarly, I often ask about special treats the child has received recently.

In this first stage it is important that the parents, not the child or the therapist, actually write down the list of routine rewards and special treats. This is a therapist demand that concretely expresses the belief that the parents have a large amount of authority in the program. It tends to support the power of the parents in the family. A misbehaving child whom they can't control almost by definition has weakened their parental authority. As we shall see, this program will strengthen that authority in several ways. Having the parents serve as the official record keeper for the program is an important first step.

Two problems are frequently encountered in this first stage of the behavior modification program. First, parents may complain that they have already tried this program and it didn't work. After hearing a brief description of the failed program it quickly becomes obvious that they have not done *this* program. This program involves several aspects of behavior modification not often found in other programs, including restrictions, consistency, and a greater appreciation of family dynamics. If I am unable to persuade the parents that they have not done the same program in the past, I may say, "Well an important difference is that you have not done the program with me."

A second common complaint is the parents' concern that there is nothing rewarding for their child. The parents believe there are no rewards for which the child will work. They may have been involved with other behavior modification programs and at that time may also have insisted that there was nothing the child wanted. This program offers two potential solutions to this challenge. First, most children want their routine rewards, and often the loss of all routine rewards has not been on the negotiating table with other programs. Second, it is the therapist's responsibility to develop with the parents and child a special treat that will "unlock the heart of the child." Skeptical parents may shake their heads in disbelief, but persistence in the quest for a reward for which the child will work has always paid off. I'm only partially joking when I explain that "every child has his price."

Two examples are a petulant eight-year-old female who decided to go along with the program so as to continue her horseback riding lessons and a rebellious 14-year-old who agreed to the program so as to have the opportunity to ride his dirt bike at a dirt bike track.

The program largely excludes material rewards for several reasons: material rewards are expensive, they take up lots of space, and they can only be used as a reward one time. Interpersonal or skill-development rewards have several advantages: they can be used over and over, and they can be used to promote the psychological development of the patient. They may enhance family functioning as well. A child whose most cherished reward is to go fishing with a parent is a perfect example of the many functions of a well-chosen interpersonal reward. It promotes closeness between parent and child, it gives the child the opportunity to learn a skill, and it can repeatedly serve as a reward. Having a sleepover, going on a family outing to a park, or going to a birthday party all serve important developmental goals for children.

Gaining the cooperation of the child by developing a list of sought-after rewards or special treats is the critical goal of this first stage of the program.

STAGE II: MISBEHAVIOR LIST

The second stage of the program, Misbehavior List, is also done in a family meeting. The behaviors are listed in a matter-of-fact tone of voice devoid of anger toward the child. It might be imagined that most children would feel accused or blamed during this session and would become upset. Surprisingly, it is rare for children to become openly distressed during this session. Some children will even help out by contributing additional misbehaviors to the list, a welcome sign that they are supporting the program. At the end of the session the child should be praised for sitting through the session and behaving well during this difficult phase of the program.

Some parents may be reluctant to mention all of the child's misbehaviors. They may feel that they are protecting the child, or they may feel embarrassed themselves by the extent of the child's misbehavior. It is important to include all of the child's misbehaviors in the program. The therapist, based on previous meetings with the family, may know that the child is misbehaving in many ways that the parents have not listed. The parents should be asked to list these other behaviors.

It is desirable to have a lot of frequently occurring misbehaviors in the behavior problem list. As was said earlier, a behavior that occurs rarely is more difficult to change than is a behavior that occurs several times a day.

STAGE III: BASELINE DATA

In the third stage, Baseline Data, a chart is constructed to record the child's misbehaviors. The left margin vertically lists all the child's misbehaviors, and the days of the week appear horizontally at the top of the chart. A mark is made each time the child engages in a listed misbehavior. The chart is usually posted in a place where the child can see it easily, such as the refrigerator. If the child rips the chart from the refrigerator the parent should keep the chart without posting it until the behavior of tearing the chart can be addressed. Those children who are likely to dispute every recorded infraction are encouraged to rein in their combative temperament by the therapist placing the parents in absolute control of deciding when an infraction is recorded. There can be no discussion between a parent and child about the fairness of giving a mark for misbehavior. This rule eliminates bickering and disputes between parents and the child patient. It also increases parental authority in the home.

Recorded behaviors are limited to observable behaviors such as cursing, not doing homework, and kicking the dog. More subtle behaviors reflecting attitude such as smirking and eye rolling do not count. As long as the child complies with the parents' demands for a specific behavior, the attitude that accompanies the requested behavior is irrelevant. It is the behavior that counts. Attitude is too vague, fleeting, and open to possible dispute to count as a misbehavior. As the child succeeds in the program, the child's attitude inevitably improves without it having to be addressed.

The misbehaviors are unweighted. A minor rule violation counts as much as a serious rule violation. One reason the program works is its simplicity; attempting to assign weights to rule violations complicates the program too much. Similarly, the program does not count positive behaviors. As the patient quickly improves with the program there is often a dramatic increase in positive behaviors reported by the parents. Recording positive behaviors and attempting to balance between positive behaviors and negative behaviors would also excessively complicate the program. Positive behaviors don't offset negative behaviors. The children should not have negative behaviors. Helping someone across the street is a commendable behavior, but it does not compensate for teasing a younger sister at home later in the day.

A question often arises about how to count repeated refusals to comply with a request. For example, if the child refuses to clean up his or her room after having been repeatedly asked to do so, should this count as one misbehavior ("refusing to clean room") or several misbehaviors ("refusing to clean room" and "not following directions")?

It should be counted as several misbehaviors. At a minimum, one day of the baseline week should have at least 10 to 20 misbehaviors. Some children dramatically improve their behavior simply as a result of the parental monitoring at the baseline data week. I am always delighted to have such a result and continue with the implementation stage to ensure that the child receives ample rewards for the behavior improvement.

Sometimes families return after the baseline week with a low rate of recorded misbehaviors, and this must be discussed further with the parents. The child's high rate of misbehaviors may have indeed improved with the careful monitoring and scrutiny of the parents, but it is also possible that the parent may not have recorded the misbehaviors. One common reason I've seen is the parents' wish to avoid open conflict with the child. It is up to the therapist to remind the parents of the necessity of accurate recording of misbehaviors.

The third stage, Baseline Data, comes to an end after a week of acceptable baseline data gathering. No rewards or loss of rewards are given as a result of gathered baseline data.

STAGE IV: IMPLEMENTATION

The fourth stage, Implementation, begins when the schedule of rewards and restrictions for misbehaviors is announced. It is important that the child not be told of the system for translating misbehaviors to restrictions until the third stage, Baseline Data, has ended. The delay creates an air of suspense and intensifies the family's involvement in the program.

Even if the total of misbehaviors for a day is 75, the schedule of misbehaviors and rewards described earlier is followed: four misbehaviors constitute a "bad" day, three misbehaviors an "okay" day, and two or fewer misbehaviors a "good" day. Many parents and therapists are tempted to have a large number of misbehaviors in a day translate into a larger number of allowable misbehaviors for an okay day or a good day. For example, if, during the Baseline Week, the total number of misbehaviors for a day were 75, perhaps for such a child it might seem more realistic to define an okay day as one that includes 10 misbehaviors. This slow "shaping" approach is unnecessary with most patients and should rarely be used as it unnecessarily slows the program down. The rare situations in which the number of misbehaviors for an okay day might be negotiated upward are discussed below.

The Implementation stage is the pay-off for everyone's hard work and can be gratifying for all those involved. But everyone should also be prepared for the first bad day of four or more misbehaviors. On that day, the child has not only failed to earn a point for a special treat but has lost all routine rewards. As stated earlier, routine rewards are daily activities that the child finds pleasurable, such as watching TV, playing outside after school, listening to music, playing electronic games, spending time on the computer, or talking on a cell phone. Children find it difficult to lose these activities for even a day, and parents may find they have to exert an effort within themselves to enforce the program. It's important to keep in mind that this program is intended to greatly limit the number of bad days—often one is all that is necessary for the child to understand that the parents are determined to enforce the restriction of privileges entailed by such a day.

Bad days usually strike early in the program. There should never be more than two bad days a week; if there is a third within a week I regard it as a crisis and meet with the family within 24 hours. Often there has been some misunderstanding about the program that may have led to an excessive number of bad days. Sometimes the child manages to find rewards despite the restrictions and thus avoids the consequences of deprivation of routinely rewarding activities. For example, a child might be confined to his or her room on a bad day, but subsequently it is learned that the room is richly furnished with diverting electronics such as satellite TV, which the child uses for endless hours of amusement. It is also possible that one parent is undermining the program, which I will explore later. If a solution cannot be found to the problem of an excessive number of bad days per week, the program might have to be abandoned.

In the crisis meeting I emphasize to the family that the program is "rigged" for the child to win. I want the child to succeed at getting his or her rewards. This is the situation in which I might give some consideration to increasing the number of permitted misbehaviors for an okay day by one or two misbehaviors if the behavior chart suggests that this is the difference between success and failure.

I estimate that 80% of children receiving the program never have a bad day. The program persuades most children to forgo misbehaving and to enjoy their newfound capacity to obtain special rewards. On the other hand, it is important for parents and therapists to be prepared for the friction that can occur with some children initially. A child may become verbally or even physically aggressive. Younger children might have to be held by the parents for a brief period of time. It is helpful to have both parents or, in single-parent homes, another adult involved at such moments. Each adult may need the psychological support as well as the physical help to implement the restraint.

From the first day of the program, management of a possible physical confrontation is kept in mind by the therapist. Efforts to avoid such a confrontation are energetically sought by winning the child over in stage one, Rewards List, as discussed above. Nonetheless, the parents' resolve to sustain a physical confrontation is developed and built during the program. This is partly done through the therapist's use of language. The family is bolstered in its resolve to set limits firmly for the child with respect to enforcing the program. I will explain, "You may have to have a fight with your child; you may have to struggle with your child." Or, "Now, while your child is small, you will be able to win the struggle. But when your child is older the outcome of the struggle will be more uncertain." The purpose of these statements is to prepare the parents and child to withstand the possible unpleasant confrontations that may initially characterize the bad day portion of the Implementation phase of the program.

Another technique I sometimes use to increase the willingness of the parents to employ the withdrawal of all rewards following a bad day is "soft restraint." This is a family therapy technique that entails the therapist asking the family not to engage in a treatment intervention because they are "not yet ready" to do the intervention. Applied to parents who waver in their resolve to withhold usual rewards, I let the parents know they aren't "ready" to carry out this phase of the program. This serves to increase the family's interest and motivation to participate in the program.

The child's age is an important consideration. Behavior modification programs are most successful for preschool and elementary school aged children. They can work in adolescents, but they are successful less often. With adolescents, there is much less control of all the reinforcers than there is in the school aged child's life. Physical restraint such as holding should not be used as a tactic in adolescents as part of this program. Adolescents are too strong, and a physical confrontation can have consequences that we all want to avoid, such as someone getting hurt. If the adolescent seems to be inviting physical confrontation, the program should be abandoned and a different strategy should be sought.

An issue that frequently arises is management of the patient's siblings. Untreated siblings sometimes become envious of the rewards the treated sibling is receiving. Often the untreated siblings are much better behaved than the treated sibling but want the program so as to receive the special treats the program affords. I am always happy to enroll the untreated siblings into the program. It reinforces the role of the program in the family and can be used as an opportunity to praise the family for successfully instituting the program. A closely related measure of program success is the parents' request to use the program on a misbehaving sibling. There is no reason that two parallel programs cannot occur in the same household.

For children whose primary arena of misbehavior is the school, it is very desirable to have the school participate as well. If the school does not participate, there is a risk that a child with a bad day at school and a good day at home will receive rewards at home, and from a reinforcement point of view, would be rewarded for misbehaving at school on that particular day. For a child with behavioral problems at school, the school must participate or the program will not work.

The program for school is the same as that for home, but in a classroom setting. I meet with the teachers and ask them to develop a list of misbehaviors while simultaneously meeting with the parents and child to develop a list of regular rewards and special treats. Then I have the teachers meet with the parents and child to review the child's lists of misbehaviors. The child brings home a simplified report card listing the number of misbehaviors, and the parents deliver the routine rewards and special treats to the child at home. Parents can offer a much richer set of rewards for the child than can the school. The school might offer extra time on the computer or extra time in recess, but typically these are small rewards compared to the special treats and routine rewards that the parents can offer.

FAMILY THERAPY CONSIDERATIONS

In the hands of a therapist there are a number of techniques to get through rough spots of the behavior therapy. Using family therapy is one such technique. Family therapy concerns the roles different members of the family may come to play in how they interact with each other. Family therapy principles are often ignored with behavior modification programs in children but can be used to enhance the success rates of the programs.

In using a family therapy approach, the therapist is doing two things at the same time. First, the therapist is helping the family begin a behavior modification intervention for the disruptive child. Second, the therapist is working with the forces in the family that help or hinder the success of the program. All behavior modification programs for children entangle the therapist with family issues. This program asks the therapist to be aware of these forces and at times to use them to enhance achieving treatment goals.

When the therapist makes a child-rearing recommendation such as this behavior modification program, he or she is often unwittingly entering into an alliance with one parent against the other. People usually do not choose life partners because of their child-rearing beliefs and are often surprised to learn once they have children that their views are discrepant on how child-rearing issues should be managed. One parent may take a tougher stance on the child's misbehavior, while the other may take a more sympathetic stance. The parents may be silent about this and content to let the therapist confirm one parent's viewpoint on child rearing and discredit the other parent's. The therapist's failure to realize and manage this may undermine the success of the program.

Furthermore, serious parental relationship difficulties may be fought out on the battlefield of child-rearing strategies. Parents who disagree about sex, love, money, and in-laws may make an effort to recruit the child as an ally in the ongoing conflict. It is important for the therapist to encourage the parents to agree on the child-rearing approach embodied by the behavior modification program regardless of other disagreements they may have. I regularly work with divorced parents who are able to come together in the interest of their child and implement the program successfully. Nonetheless, there may be family situations so conflicted that implementation of this program is not possible.

Family dynamics are a central element in planning the entire treatment; the therapist must attempt to understand the structure of the family and his or her own role in its structure. A typical structure in families with a disruptive child is that the child has equal or more power than the parents. The child's misbehavior usurps the parents' authority. The family therapist initially enters the family with more power than the parents or child. The therapist starts to tell family members to do things such as make lists, record behaviors, etc., and the family begins to listen. The parents make the lists, record behaviors, dispense rewards, and enforce restrictions and in this way gain their rightful authority in the family. This is the family structure the therapist seeks to develop.

At the end of the therapy there will be one last change in the family structure: the therapist must extract himself or herself from the family. Because the therapist has been planning to leave the family and has focused every intervention on strengthening the parents from the first session of the behavior modification program, he or she can leave the family with relative ease. The parents know how to run the program and have little further need for the therapist (Minuchin, 1974).

The behavior modification program uses a family therapy technique known as the "family task." A family task is a request made by the therapist to a family member to do something. In the program described here, the therapist asks the parents and child to engage in a variety of activities such as making lists and rewarding the child. Whenever someone is asked to do something, it creates an opportunity for the therapist to learn something about the person of whom the request is made. If the parent or child complies with the request, this demonstrates at a minimum ability and willingness to comply. If the parent or child does not perform the requested task, the therapist can explore the reasons for the failure to comply. This creates a pathway for the therapist to explore family functioning and/or individual functioning. The case of Jasmine and her parents, below, illustrates a therapist's exploration of a family's inability to perform the task of withholding routine rewards following a bad day.

Jasmine was a bright, verbal 11-year-old girl whose incorrigible and intense misbehavior had failed to respond to medication or behavioral interventions. The family was sent to me for behavior modification therapy. Using the procedures described above, lists of routine rewards, special treats and misbehaviors were generated by the parents. Her teachers supplied an additional misbehavior list. During the Baseline Data phase, 168 misbehaviors per day were recorded. The program was implemented with the teachers sending home the number of daily misbehaviors and the parents rewarding or restricting Jasmine based on her behavior at school.

On the first day of the program Jasmine received four misbehaviors. This was a great improvement from her previous high level of misbehaviors per day but was, according to the rules of the program, a bad day. Jasmine lost all of her routine rewards the next day. For Jasmine, this meant spending most of the time after returning home from school in her room except for dinner and some family time. It also meant no dessert. Following this day of no routine rewards, Jasmine's misbehavior frequency dropped to two misbehaviors per day (a good day with a point for a special treat) and remained there.

In the session immediately before the implementation of the program the mother, in the presence of the father, confided that Jasmine's misbehavior had led her to feel as if she had failed as a mother. Jasmine's defiance quickly reduced the mother to tears, and she often cried in front of Jasmine. The father was quiet during his wife's recitation. After Jasmine's dramatic improvement, the father began to boast that he had attempted to sabotage the restrictions. He had snuck various desserts and candies into Jasmine's room during the evening. He complained that his wife was too tough on Jasmine. He bemoaned her lack of sympathy for her daughter's difficulties.

Jasmine's father later related that he had been abused and deprived by an alcoholic father and had resolved to ensure a happy childhood for his own child by providing numerous pleasures and rewards. Jasmine's mother confided that her own father had been a violent alcoholic and that Jasmine's rages reminded her of her father and made it particularly difficult for her to set limits for Jasmine.

Initially, in this case it appeared as if the mother would have the most difficulty implementing the program because of her tearful appearance and complaints of helplessness in dealing with Jasmine. Unexpectedly, it was father who experienced the greatest internal obstacles with the limit-setting tasks of the program. The task of depriving Jasmine of routine rewards and the parents' difficulties with the task led them to disclose in a highly affectively charged manner elements of their own childhoods directly related to their difficulties in effective limit setting for Jasmine. This enabled them to be more comfortable and more effective with enforcing the restrictive aspects of the program (Kaplan, 1979).

FOR PARENTS ONLY

There are some things you need to know before trying the program.

First, if your child has ADHD, get him or her treated for it successfully with medication.

Second, if your child is in treatment with any doctors or therapists, obtain their permission to use the program.

Third, be sure to enlist the support you need. If there is another adult in your home with whom you are raising your child, establish agreement to try to implement the program together.

Fourth, you *must* involve a therapist or other professional if your child has violent temper tantrums or assaultive behavior, if more than two bad days in a week occur once the program has begun, or if the program does not seem to have worked after four weeks of implementation.

REFERENCES

Kaplan, S. L. (1979). Behavior modification as a task in the family therapy of a disruptive child. *J Am Ac Child Psychiatry*, *18*(3), 492–504.

Minuchin, S. (1974). *Families and family therapy*. Cambridge: Harvard University Press.

Afterword

The rich diversity of cultures created by humankind is a testament to our ability to develop and adapt in diverse ways. But however varied different cultures may be, children are not endlessly malleable; they all share basic psychological and physical needs that must be met to ensure healthy development. The Childhood in America series examines the extent to which American culture meets children's irreducible needs. Without question, many children growing up in the United States lead privileged lives. They have been spared the ravages of war, poverty, malnourishment, sexism, and racism. However, despite our nation's resources, not all children share these privileges. Additionally, values that are central to American culture, such as self-reliance, individualism, privacy of family life, and consumerism, have created a climate in which parenting has become intolerably labor-intensive, and children are being taxed beyond their capacity for healthy adaptation. Record levels of psychiatric disturbance, violence, poverty, apathy, and despair among our children speak to our current cultural crisis.

Although our elected officials profess their commitment to "family values," policies that support family life are woefully lacking and inferior to those in other industrialized nations. American families are burdened by inadequate parental leave, a health care system that does not provide universal coverage for children, a minimum wage that is not a living wage, "welfare to work" policies that require parents to leave their children for long stretches of time, unregulated and inadequately subsidized daycare, an unregulated entertainment industry that exposes children to sex and violence, and a two-tiered public education system that delivers inferior education to poor children and frequently ignores individual differences in learning styles and profiles of intelligence. As a result, many families are taxed to the breaking point. In addition, our fascination with technological innovation is creating a family lifestyle that is dominated by screens rather than human interaction.

The Childhood in America series seeks out leading childhood experts from across the disciplines to promote dialogue, research, and understanding regarding how best to raise and educate psychologically healthy children to ensure that they will acquire the wisdom, heart, and courage needed to make choices for the betterment of society.

Sharna Olfman, PhD
Series Editor
Childhood in America

Index

Adderall XR (mixed amphetamine salts extended release), 137
ADHD. *See* Attention deficit hyperactivity disorder
Adolescent bipolar disorder, 83–88; aggression and misdiagnosis of, 85–86; features, 86–88; manic symptoms in adolescents, 83–85. *See also* Adult bipolar disorder; Bipolar disorder; Pediatric bipolar disorder
Adolescents: behavior modification programs for, 168; importance of studying separately from children, 126; manic symptoms in, 83–85; romantic love in, 84–85; stimulant use by, 133, 143; turmoil in, 88. *See also* Adolescent bipolar disorder; Child and adolescent depression
Adult bipolar disorder: depression in, 7–8, 82; diagnosis of, 8; hypomania in, 4–5; lithium for, 95, 96–97; mania in, 4–7; pediatric bipolar disorder compared to, 15–16; risperidone for, 101; treatment, 23. *See also* Adolescent bipolar disorder; Bipolar disorder; Pediatric bipolar disorder
Age of onset: family studies, 43–46; self-report, 46–48
Aggression: antipsychotics for, 103, 155–56; misdiagnosis of bipolar disorder in adolescents and, 85–86; stimulants for, 130
Ambition, and grandiosity, 31
American Heart Association, 141
"Americanization of Mental Illness, The" (Watters), 56, 57–58
Amish children, 44–46
Angell, Marcia, 109
Anger, 15–16, 20
Anorexia nervosa, 57–58
Anticonvulsants, 97–98. *See also* Valproate (Depakote)
Antidepressants, 81–82, 144
Antipsychotics: as aggression treatment, 103, 155–56; first-generation, 99–100; increase in use of, 102, 103; second-generation, 100–103; side effects, 99–100, 156
Anxiety, in play therapy, 76
Attention deficit hyperactivity disorder (ADHD): in adults, 10; as

About the Series Editor
and Advisers

SHARNA OLFMAN, PhD, series editor, is a clinical psychologist and Professor of Psychology in the Department of Humanities at Point Park University. Her books include *The Sexualization of Childhood* (2008), *Bipolar Children* (2007), *Child Honoring: How To Turn This World Around* (co-edited with Raffi Cavoukian, 2006), *Childhood Lost . . . How American Culture Is Failing Our Kids* (2005), and *All Work and No Play . . . How Educational Reforms Are Harming Our Preschoolers* (2004). Dr. Olfman is a partner in the Alliance for Childhood and a member of the Council of Human Development.

JOAN ALMON is Coordinator of the U.S. branch of the Alliance for Childhood and Co-Chair of the Waldorf Early Childhood Association of North America. She is internationally renowned as consultant to Waldorf educators and training programs, and she is the author of numerous articles on Waldorf education.

JANE M. HEALY has appeared on most major media in the United States and is frequently consulted regarding the effects of new technologies on the developing brain. She holds a PhD in educational psychology from Case Western University and has done postdoctoral work in developmental neuropsychology. Formerly on the faculties of Cleveland State University and John Carroll University, she is internationally recognized as a lecturer and a consultant with many years experience as a classroom teacher, reading/learning specialist, and elementary administrator. She is author of numerous articles as well as the books *Endangered Minds: Why Our Children Don't Think and What We Can Do About It* (1999), *How to Have an Intelligent and Creative Conversation with Your Kids* (1994), *Your Child's Growing Mind: A Guide to Learning and Brain Development from Birth to Adolescence* (1994), and *Failure to Connect: How Computers Affect Our Children's Minds—For Better or Worse* (1998).

STUART SHANKER, PhD Oxon, is a distinguished Professor of Philosophy and Psychology at York University in Toronto. He is, with Stanley Greenspan, Co-Director of the Council of Human Development and Associate Chair for Canada of the Interdisciplinary Council of Learning and Developmental Disorders. He has won numerous awards and currently holds grants from the Unicorn Foundation, the Templeton Foundation, and Cure Autism Now. His books include *The First Idea: How Symbols, Language, and Intelligence Evolved from Our Primate Ancestors to Modern Humans* (2004), *Toward a Psychology of Global Interdependency* (2002), and *Wittgenstein's Remarks on the Foundations of Animal Intelligence* (1998).

MEREDITH F. SMALL, PhD, is a writer and Professor of Anthropology at Cornell University. Trained as a primate behaviorist, she now writes about all areas of anthropology, natural history, and health. Besides numerous publications in academic journals, Dr. Small contributes regularly to *Discover* and *New Scientist*, and she is a commentator on National Public Radio's *All Things Considered*. She is the author of five books including *What's Love Got to Do With It? The Evolution of Human Mating* (1996), *Our Babies, Ourselves; How Biology and Culture Shape the Way We Parent* (1999), and *Kids: How Biology and Culture Shape the Way We Parent* (2001; paperback, 2002). Dr. Small is currently working on a book about the anthropology of mental health titled *The Culture of Our Discontent* in which she explores the now standard medical model of mental illness with the causes and cures of "abnormal" behavior in traditional cultures.

About the Author

STUART L. KAPLAN, MD, is a practicing child psychiatrist with over 40 years of experience treating children, adolescents, and their families. He is a Clinical Professor of Psychiatry at the Penn State College of Medicine and has been the Director of Child and Adolescent Psychiatry and Director of Child Psychiatry Training at university medical schools. He is a Distinguished Life Fellow of the American Academy of Child and Adolescent Psychiatry. Dr. Kaplan has authored more than 100 scientific journal articles and presentations at national and international professional meetings. He has served on the editorial board of the *Journal of the American Academy of Child and Adolescent Psychiatry*, the *Journal of Child and Adolescent Psychopharmacology*, and the *Hillside Journal of Clinical Psychiatry*.